The Diabetic Way

Everyday recipes for the Diabetic

A book would not be complete without a few thank yous...

... To my husband, Henry Halmon, who inspired me, helped me and ate my many mistakes. I owe a debt of love and gratitude to him forever.

... To Amy Ludzig, chef and great typist, thank you for being "Recipe Editor" and assistant, and for all your hard work.

... To Dr. Louis Train, Sr., M.D., thank you for all your help, research and support on finding an alternative ingredient to make a diabetic's life so much easier.

... And to Virginia and George Uppencamp who were most instrumental in inspiring me to create a diabetic cookbook and encouraged me to look for something new. Without your inspiration, this book would never have happened. Your help and friendship means a lot to me and I thank you from the bottom of my heart.

...To Gary and Donna Cowart, thanks for all the help you have done for me with electrical work and kindness to my husband. Donna has always been so kind to us every time I called and needed something, she got Gary to come and fix it! God Bless You Both.

... To Allen Williams at Randalls on Holcombe at Buffalo Speedway, thank you for your kindness and help, time and time again.

... To Joe at La Madeleine French Bakery & Cafe in the Village, thank you so much for everything. You've been extremely helpful, kind and supportive.

... And to all the vendors who have supported this project and sent samples. A big Texas thank you!

If I have forgotten someone, I apologize, but your support is greatly appreciated.

(Warning: If you eat too much of a dessert, you may have a tummy ache.)

The Diabetic Way: Everyday recipes with the Diabetic in Mind
Copyright © 1997 by MVG Cookbooks, Inc.

edited by Mary Halmon

All rights reserved. No part of this book may be reproduced in any form or by any electronic or mechanical means, including information storage and retrieval systems, without permission in writing from the publisher, except by a reviewer who may quote brief passages in a review.

Printed in the United States of America

Book design and layout by Ecoversity, Manvel, TX

Printed by Met Printing, Inc., Houston, Texas

ISBN 0-9659359-0-6

As my husband, Henry, and I reached the "golden age", diabetes became a major concern in our lives. The number of diabetic cookbooks on the market seemed slim and narrow. As someone who enjoys cooking and sharing my goodies with others, I felt there was the need for a varied cookbook designed with the diabetic in mind. Not special, unusual recipes that needed special ingredients, but those you could find on the regular grocery store shelf. This book is the result of that need. The recipes have been adapted from a variety of sources and can be used in everyday menu preparation. Including the use of a new and exciting sugar substitute, maltitol, that has been doctor researched not to raise the blood sugar in a diabetic. In a society that is aging, I hope you find this to fit the bill.

Happy cooking, the Diabetic Way!

Mary Halmon

Appetizers

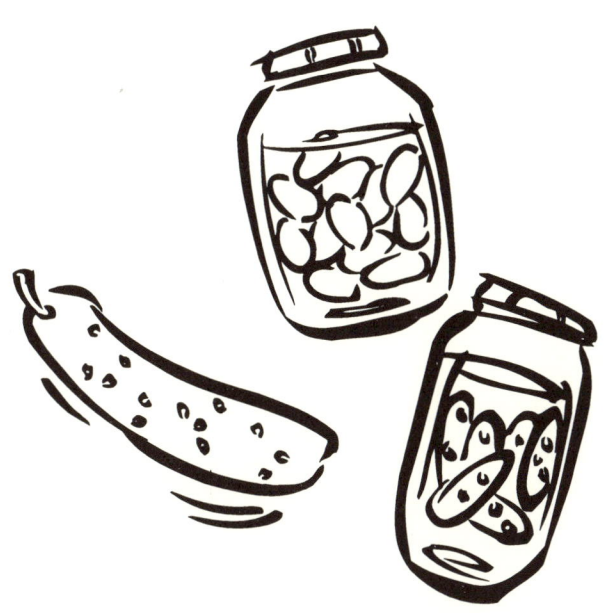

Appetizers

Artichoke Dip

Serving Size: 12

2 c. artichoke hearts, drained and chopped
2 c. sour cream, light
1 1/2 c. reduced-calorie mayonnaise
2 pkg. Hidden Valley Ranch dry salad dressing mix
Garlic powder to taste
Lemon juice to taste

Mix all ingredients well and refrigerate. Serve with toast points or french bread rounds.

Per serving: 108 Calories; 9g Fat (70% calories from fat); 2g Protein; 7g Carbohydrate; 13mg Cholesterol; 188mg Sodium

Artichoke Dip 2

Serving Size: 6

20 oz. artichoke hearts, frozen
1 c. fat-free mayonnaise
1 c. fat-free Parmesan cheese
6 cloves garlic, minced
fat-free Parmesan cheese to taste

Cook artichokes according to package directions without salt or fat. Drain and cut artichokes into small pieces. Blend artichokes with mayonnaise, cheese and garlic. Place the mixture in baking dish that has been prepared with nonstick cooking spray. Bake at 350°F for 20 minutes or until hot and bubbly. Sprinkle the top with Parmesan cheese. Serve with fat-free crackers or fresh vegetables.

Per serving: 131 Calories; less than one gram Fat (1% calories from fat); 10g Protein; 26g Carbohydrate; 16mg Cholesterol; 741mg Sodium

Artichoke Heart Spread

Serving Size: 4

8 oz. artichoke hearts, drained and chopped
1 can fat-free Parmesan cheese, grated
1/2 c. fat-free sour cream
1/2 c. fat-free mayonnaise
8 oz. fat-free cream cheese
1/4 tsp. minced garlic
2 jalapenos, seeded & chopped

Mix all ingredients together until smooth. Put in ovenproof dish that has been prepared with nonstick cooking spray. Bake at 350°F for 30 to 45 minutes or until lightly brown on top. Serve with fat-free crackers or toasted sourdough bread slices.

Per serving: 131 Calories; less than one gram Fat (1% calories from fat); 13g Protein; 21g Carbohydrate; 14mg Cholesterol; 805mg Sodium

Artichoke Pita Chips

Serving Size: 60

1/4 c. water
9 oz. artichoke hearts, frozen
1 c. celery thinly, sliced
2 green onions, sliced
1 c. nonfat cottage cheese
1/3 c. fat-free mayonnaise
1 tbsp. lemon juice
8 small pita bread
 grated fat-free Parmesan cheese, optional

Combine artichokes, water and celery in small saucepan. Simmer, covered for 15 minutes. Drain. Combine artichoke mixture and onions in food processor and chop finely. Place in large bowl. Puree cottage cheese in processor. Add the pureed cottage cheese, mayonnaise and lemon juice to the artichoke mixture in the large bowl. Mix well. Split pitas in half and spread 3 tablespoons of artichoke mixture inside each one. Sprinkle with cheese if desired. Cut each half into 4 wedges. Arrange on cookie sheet that has been prepared with nonstick cooking spray. Bake at 400°F for 10 to 15 minutes or until the edges of the pita bread turns brown. Serve immediately.

Per serving: 29 Calories; less than one gram Fat (3% calories from fat); 1g Protein; 6g Carbohydrate; 0mg Cholesterol; 76mg Sodium

Baked Fried Zucchini and Mushrooms

Serving Size: 8

2 large zucchini
16 fresh mushrooms
1/2 c. egg substitute
1 c. corn flake crumbs
garlic powder to taste
onion powder to taste

Wash zucchini and slice into 1/2 to 3/4 inch thick slices. Pour egg substitute into 1 bowl. Mix corn flake crumbs, garlic powder and onion powder together in another bowl. Dip zucchini and mushrooms in egg and then into corn flake crumb mixture coating all sides. Place on cookie sheet that has been lined with foil. Bake at 400°F for 15 to 20 minutes or until crispy and vegetables are cooked.
Serving Ideas: Serve with fat-free honey mustard or ranch dressing

---

Per serving: 77 Calories; 2g Fat (21% calories from fat); 4g Protein; 12g Carbohydrate; 0mg Cholesterol; 152mg Sodium

Billie Jo's Chicken Wings

Serving Size: 12

3 1/2 lbs. chicken wings, cut
Salt to taste
Pepper to taste
Garlic powder to taste
1 tbsp. lemon juice
3 tbsps. Sugar Twin brown sugar replacement
1/4 c. low sodium soy sauce
5 tbsps. maltitol
6 peppercorns, whole
1 c. hot water

Cut wings in half and discard the tips. Rinse and pat dry. Place in 2 quart glass casserole dish. Sprinkle with salt, pepper and garlic powder. In separate bowl, mix rest of ingredients. Pour over wings. Cover with foil and bake at 350°F for 2 hours. Remove foil, baste. Lower temperature to 300°F and bake an additional 30 minutes. Baste.

Per serving: 185 Calories; 12g Fat (54% calories from fat); 14g Protein; 8g Carbohydrate; 55mg Cholesterol; 254mg Sodium

Black Bean Dip

Serving Size: 8

1 tbsp. green chilies, chopped
1/4 c. onion, chopped
1 clove garlic, minced
15 oz. black beans, cooked and drained
1/2 c. low-fat sour cream
1/2 tsp. ground cumin
1/4 tsp. salt
2 tbsps. cilantro, chopped

Place chilies, onion, garlic, and beans in a blender or food processor and blend until almost smooth. Stir in sour cream, cumin, cilantro and salt. Serve cold or slowly heat up in a heavy sauce pot if you would like to serve it warm.

Per serving: 93 Calories; 1g Fat (10% calories from fat); 6g Protein; 15g Carbohydrate; 3mg Cholesterol; 86mg Sodium

Black Bean Dip 2

Serving Size: 4

2 c. black beans, cooked and drained
4 tsps. tomato sauce
3 tbsps. water
1 clove garlic, minced
2 tsps. lemon juice
2 green onion, chopped fine

Rinse beans. Combine beans, tomato sauce, water, garlic and lemon juice in food processor or blender. Process approximately 1 minute or until smooth paste forms. Pour into serving bowl and top with green onions. Serve with fat-free crackers.

Per serving: 357 Calories; 2g Fat (4% calories from fat); 22g Protein; 67g Carbohydrate; 0mg Cholesterol; 48mg Sodium

Caponata

Serving Size: 8

1 c. red bell pepper, chopped
1/2 c. onion, chopped
2 cloves garlic, minced
2 tbsps. extra virgin olive oil
7 c. eggplant, peeled and chopped
3/4 c. tomato, chopped
2 tsps. dried basil
2 tbsps. balsamic vinegar
1/4 tsp. salt
1/4 tsp. pepper

Cook onion over medium heat with olive oil in a large skillet until the onion is soft. Add garlic, then cook for one minute. Add tomatoes and eggplant. Cook 8-10 minutes, stirring frequently, until the eggplant is very soft. Stir in remaining ingredients. Cover and refrigerate until completely cooled.

This recipe is great as an appetizer when served with crackers or chunks of fresh french bread.

Per serving: 55 Calories; 4g Fat (54% calories from fat); 1g Protein; 6g Carbohydrate; 0mg Cholesterol; 69mg Sodium

Cheese and Artichoke Dip

Serving Size: 12

24 oz. bread round loaf
1/4 lb. reduced-calorie margarine
5 green onions, chopped
12 cloves fresh garlic, finely minced
8 oz. fat-free cream cheese, room temperature
16 oz. fat-free sour cream
12 oz. low-fat Cheddar cheese, grated
10 oz. artichoke hearts, drained and chopped
Wheat Thins® crackers

Cut 5 inch hole in top of bread. Remove soft bread of top and reserve crust. Scoop out most of bread inside. Saute green onions and 6 cloves of garlic in 2 tablespoons margarine until soft. Cut cream cheese into small pieces, and add to green onions. Add sour cream and Cheddar cheese. Mix well. Fold in artichoke hearts. Pour mixture into hollowed out bread. Put top on and wrap in heavy aluminum foil. Bake at 350°F for 1 1/2 to 2 hours or until heat thoroughly. To serve, remove foil and serve with low-fat Wheat Thins.

Per serving: 341 Calories; 11g Fat (28% calories from fat); 21g Protein; 44g Carbohydrate; 22mg Cholesterol; 733mg Sodium

Cold Veggie Platter

Serving Size: 12

16 oz. beets, small
1 lb. cauliflower florets, cooked and chilled
1 lb. baby carrots, cooked and chilled
1 lb. green beans, cooked and chilled
1 c. fat-free mayonnaise
1/2 c. fat-free sour cream
2 tbsps. lemon juice
1 tsp. salt substitute
1/2 c. frozen chopped spinach, thawed and drained

Blend mayonnaise, sour cream, lemon juice, salt substitute and spinach together until smooth and creamy. Refrigerate several hours or overnight. To prepare platter, arrange cooked vegetables on serving plate and serve with sauce as a dip.
Notes: Fresh vegetables make this dish especially delicious!

Per serving: 71 Calories; less than one gram Fat (4% calories from fat); 3g Protein; 16g Carbohydrate; 1mg Cholesterol; 315mg Sodium

Corned Beef and Cheese Dip

Serving Size: 12

2 jars dried beef, chopped
8 oz. fat-free Cheddar cheese
1/4 c. pimiento, chopped
1 can tomatoes, chopped
1 c. fat-free mayonnaise

Mix ingredients together. Bake at 325°F for 15 minutes.

Per serving: 55 Calories; less than one gram Fat (3% calories from fat); 8g Protein; 6g Carbohydrate; 5mg Cholesterol; 554mg Sodium

Crab Appetizer

Serving Size: 6

12 oz. fat-free cream cheese
12 oz. cocktail sauce for seafood
8 oz. crab surimi seafood chunks (artificial crab)

Soften cream cheese. Layer cream cheese on serving dish, cover with cocktail sauce. Break up crabmeat into small pieces and crumble over cocktail sauce. Serve at room temperature with fat-free crackers.

Per serving: 138 Calories; 1g Fat (4% calories from fat); 15g Protein; 17g Carbohydrate; 22mg Cholesterol; 854mg Sodium

Crab Devils

Serving Size: 6

1 pkg. crab surimi seafood chunks, drained
3/4 c. fat-free mayonnaise
1/2 c. fat-free Parmesan cheese
1/2 tsp. Worcestershire sauce
Tabasco sauce to taste
onion powder to taste
pimiento strips for garnish
parsley for garnish
fat-free onion crackers

Combine crabmeat, mayonnaise, cheese, Worcestershire sauce, Tabasco and onion powder. Mix well. Spread on onion crackers. Sprinkle with extra Parmesan cheese. Broil until lightly browned and bubbly. Cool slightly. Garnish with pimento strips and parsley, if desired.

Per serving: 53 Calories; less than one gram Fat (1% calories from fat); 4g Protein; 10g Carbohydrate; 9mg Cholesterol; 463mg Sodium

Crab Spread

Serving Size: 6

1 lb. lump crabmeat, picked over
2 tbsps. fresh lemon juice
2 tbsps. low-fat sour cream
1/4 c. low-fat mayonnaise
1/2 tsp. dried dill
1/4 tsp. celery salt
1/2 c. bell pepper, minced
1/4 c. red onion, minced
2 tsps. minced garlic

In a medium bowl, toss crab with lemon juice. Add remaining ingredients and mix well. Serve with crackers or garlic toast.

Notes: Whenever you purchase crabmeat already torn from the crab, it is a good idea to pick through the meat to make sure no hard pieces of cartilage remain.

Per serving: 108 Calories; 4g Fat (32% calories from fat); 14g Protein; 4g Carbohydrate; 63mg Cholesterol; 341mg Sodium

Crabmeat Dip

Serving Size: 4

8 oz. fat-free cream cheese
8 oz. crab surimi seafood chunks
1 c. ketchup, low sodium
1/4 c. horseradish
1/2 tsp. parsley
fat-free crackers

Combine ketchup and horseradish in small bowl, set aside. Spread cream cheese on serving dish, top with crabmeat and cover with ketchup. Garnish with parsley.

Per serving: 184 Calories; 1g Fat (4% calories from fat); 18g Protein; 26g Carbohydrate; 27mg Cholesterol; 452mg Sodium

Creamy Salsa

Serving Size: 4

4 oz. fat-free cream cheese
1/3 c. salsa, thick and chunky
 pepper to taste

Beat cream cheese in small bowl until creamy and smooth. Add salsa and pepper. Mix well. To serve, spread over warm fat-free toast.

Per serving: 31 Calories; less than one gram Fat (10% calories from fat); 4g Protein; 2g Carbohydrate; 5mg Cholesterol; 315mg Sodium

Curry Dip

Serving Size: 4

1/2 c. fat-free sour cream
1 c. fat-free mayonnaise
1 clove garlic, crushed
2 tsps. lemon juice
4 tsps. Sugar Twin brown sugar replacement
1 tbsp. curry powder
1/2 c. parsley, finely minced

Mix all ingredients and chill. Serve with fresh vegetables.

Per serving: 95 Calories; 1g Fat (4% calories from fat); 4g Protein; 22g Carbohydrate; 3mg Cholesterol; 817mg Sodium

Dill Dip

Serving Size: 5

1 c. low-fat sour cream
3 tbsps. low-fat mayonnaise
2 tbsps. green onions with tops, sliced
1 tbsp. fresh dill, chopped
1/4 tsp. salt
2 tsps. fresh lemon juice
1 tsp. Dijon-style mustard

Combine all ingredients cover and refrigerate for at least one hour to allow flavors to blend. Serve as a dip for vegetables or as a sauce for fish.

Per serving: 84 Calories; 5g Fat (53% calories from fat); 3g Protein; 7g Carbohydrate; 13mg Cholesterol; 216mg Sodium

Guacamole

Serving Size: 8

3/4 c. low-fat sour cream
1 each avocado, mashed
3/4 c. tomatoes, seeded & chopped
2 tbsps. onion, chopped
2 tbsps. fresh cilantro, chopped
1 tbsp. lime juice
1 each jalapeno pepper, seeded & chopped
1 clove garlic, minced
1 dash pepper

Combine all ingredients until smooth. Cover and refrigerate. Let stand an hour before serving to allow flavors to blend.

Per serving: 66 Calories; 4g Fat (52% calories from fat); 2g Protein; 6g Carbohydrate; 4mg Cholesterol; 30mg Sodium

Honey Mustard Dip

Serving Size: 8

1/2 c. maltitol, honey flavored
1/2 c. Dijon mustard
2 tbsps. teriyaki sauce
2 tbsps. ginger root, grated
1/2 tsp. hot pepper sauce

Combine all ingredients. Blend well. Serve with fresh vegetables.

Per serving: 50 Calories; 1g Fat (9% calories from fat); 1g Protein; 14g Carbohydrate; 0mg Cholesterol; 361mg Sodium

Hot and Spicy Tomato Salsa

Serving Size: 16

3 tomatoes, chopped
15 oz. tomato puree
6 cloves garlic, minced
4 oz. jalapeno, diced
3 tbsps. onion, chopped
1/3 c. apple juice, no sugar added
1/4 can lemon juice
1/2 c. cayenne
1/2 tsp. pepper
1/4 c. fresh cilantro, chopped

Combine all ingredients except cilantro in medium saucepan. Bring to boil over high heat, stirring constantly. Reduce to medium heat and cook, uncovered 15 minutes. Stir occasionally. Add cilantro. Serve with fat-free tortilla chips.
Notes: Can be frozen up to 2 months.

Per serving: 34 Calories; 1g Fat (12% calories from fat); 1g Protein; 8g Carbohydrate; 0mg Cholesterol; 110mg Sodium

Hot Bean Dip

Serving Size: 4

32 oz. fat-free refried beans
3 c. fat-free cheddar cheese
1 c. diced tomato
1/2 c. chopped onion
4 oz. chopped green chilies

Combine beans, 2 cups cheese, tomato, onion and chilies. Mix well. Spread mixture in casserole dish that has been prepared with nonstick cooking spray and sprinkle with remaining cheese. Bake at 350°F for 25 to 30 minutes or until cheese is melted and bubbly. Serve with fat-free tortilla chips.

Per serving: 323 Calories; less than one gram Fat (1% calories from fat); 37g Protein; 43g Carbohydrate; 15mg Cholesterol; 1489mg Sodium

Hot Crab Dip

Serving Size: 12

8 oz. crab meat, flaked
3/4 c. Parmesan cheese, shredded
1 c. fat-free mayonnaise
1/2 tsp. garlic, minced
3 dashes hot pepper sauce

Combine all ingredients in medium bowl. Pour into 1 quart casserole dish that has been prepared with nonstick cooking spray. Bake, uncovered, at 350°F for 30 minutes. Sprinkle additional Parmesan cheese on top. Serve with French bread rounds or your favorite crackers.

Per serving: 58 Calories; 2g Fat (28% calories from fat); 6g Protein; 4g Carbohydrate; 21mg Cholesterol; 410mg Sodium

Mexican Layer Dip

Serving Size: 12

16 oz. fat-free refried beans
1 c. fat-free sour cream
1/2 c. fat-free mayonnaise
1 package taco seasoning mix
2 c. green onion, chopped
8 oz. chopped green chilies
2 c. chopped fresh tomatoes
10 oz. fat-free cheddar cheese, shredded

Spread beans on large platter. Mix sour cream, mayonnaise and taco seasoning together, cover beans. Sprinkle with green onions. Top with chilies and tomatoes. Spread cheese over the top. Refrigerate. Serve with fat-free tortilla chips, crackers or vegetables.

Per serving: 110 Calories; less than one gram Fat (1% calories from fat); 12g Protein; 18g Carbohydrate; 6mg Cholesterol; 656mg Sodium

Mushrooms Florentine

Serving Size: 5

10 oz. frozen chopped spinach, thawed and drained
1 c. seasoned bread stuffing
1 each egg
1 tbsp. extra virgin olive oil
1/4 c. Parmesan cheese, grated
1/2 tsp. pepper
1 tbsp. minced garlic
1 tsp. dried basil
20 large mushrooms

Preheat oven to 350°F. Combine all ingredients except mushrooms and mix well. Clean mushrooms, remove and discard the stems. Spoon stuffing evenly into each mushroom cap. Bake for 15-20 minutes, serve hot.

Notes: To wash or not to wash…that is the question. Among cooking circles there is a debate about whether it is okay to wash mushrooms with water or just brush them off with a soft towel. Granted, mushrooms do absorb water when they are washed, but the amount is so little I say wash them to get off the excess dirt.

Per serving: 178 Calories; 6g Fat (29% calories from fat); 9g Protein; 23g Carbohydrate; 40mg Cholesterol; 767mg Sodium

Nacho Cheese Dip

Serving Size: 6

8 oz. nonfat cream cheese
1 c. nonfat cheddar cheese, Mexican flavored
2 tsps. skim milk
1/2 c. picante sauce

Combine cream cheese and cheddar cheese in small saucepan. Cook over low heat until melted. Add milk and salsa. Continue cooking 10 minutes or until thoroughly heated. Serve with fat-free tortilla chips.

Per serving: 67 Calories; less than one gram Fat (5% calories from fat); 12g Protein; 3g Carbohydrate; 10mg Cholesterol; 508mg Sodium

Onion Cheese Puffs

Serving Size: 6

1 c. fat-free mayonnaise
1 c. fat-free Parmesan cheese
1/2 c. onion, grated
3/4 tbsp. skim milk

Combine all ingredients. Mix well. Spread mixture on assorted fat-free crackers and place under broiler for 2 minutes or bake at 350°F until golden brown.

Per serving: 86 Calories; 0g Fat (0% calories from fat); 7g Protein; 16g Carbohydrate; 16mg Cholesterol; 652mg Sodium

Onion Spread

Serving Size: 4

1/2 c. fat-free mayonnaise
8 oz. fat-free cream cheese
1/2 c. green onion, chopped
1 tsp. Worcestershire sauce
1/4 tsp. garlic powder

Combine mayonnaise and cream cheese. Mix well. Add remaining ingredients. Mix well. Serve with fat-free crackers.

Per serving: 79 Calories; 0g Fat (0% calories from fat); 8g Protein; 9g Carbohydrate; 10mg Cholesterol; 734mg Sodium

Oven Zucchini Fries

Serving Size: 4

1/4 c. seasoned bread crumbs
2 tbsps. grated Parmesan cheese
1/4 tsp. garlic powder
2 medium zucchini
1 tsp. extra virgin olive oil
3 tbsps. water
1 c. spaghetti sauce

Preheat oven to 475°F. Mix breadcrumbs, cheese, and garlic powder in a pie pan and set aside. Cut both zucchini lengthwise into four equal pieces, then cut them again in half crosswise. Combine zucchini, water and oil in a bowl and toss until zucchini is coated. Press zucchini into crumb mixture then lay them single layer on a baking pan that has been coated with nonstick cooking spray. Bake for 10 minutes or until golden brown. Heat spaghetti sauce and serve with zucchini sticks.

Per serving: 129 Calories; 5g Fat (36% calories from fat); 4g Protein; 17g Carbohydrate; 3mg Cholesterol; 568mg Sodium

Pepper Cheese Dip

Serving Size: 6

2 c. nonfat mozzarella cheese, shredded
2 c. American cheese, shredded
6 green onion, sliced
2/3 c. red bell pepper, chopped
2 tbsps. jalapeno, diced

Spray saucepan with cooking spray. Melt cheeses in saucepan over medium-low heat, 5 to 10 minutes. Add rest of vegetables. Serve with reduced-salt tortilla chips.

Per serving: 246 Calories; 12g Fat (43% calories from fat); 23g Protein; 14g Carbohydrate; 42mg Cholesterol; 566mg Sodium

Salmon Tortilla Appetizers

Serving Size: 24

15 oz. canned salmon, flaked
8 oz. lowfat cream cheese, softened
4 tbsps. salsa
2 tbsps. fresh parsley
1 tbsp. cilantro
1/4 tsp. ground cumin, optional
1 dash garlic powder
8 flour tortillas (8 inch)

Drain salmon and remove any bones. In a small bowl combine salmon, cream cheese, salsa, parsley and cilantro. Add cumin. Spread about 2 tablespoons mixture over each tortilla. Roll each tortilla up tightly and wrap individually with plastic wrap. Refrigerate 2-3 hours; slice each tortilla into bite-size pieces.

Per serving: 86 Calories; 4g Fat (39% calories from fat); 6g Protein; 7g Carbohydrate; 15mg Cholesterol; 238mg Sodium

Spinach and Cheese Bites

Serving Size: 24

2 eggs
6 tbsps. flour, all-purpose
1 1/2 c. lowfat cheddar cheese, shredded
10 oz. frozen spinach, thawed and drained
2 c. lowfat cottage cheese
1 pinch ground nutmeg
1 dash fresh ground black pepper
1 dash cayenne
3 tbsps. seasoned bread crumbs

Preheat oven to 350°F. In a large bowl, beat eggs with flour until smooth. Squeeze spinach to dry then add to egg mixture along with cottage cheese, cheddar cheese, pepper, cayenne, and nutmeg. Mix well. Pour into 13 x 9 x 2-inch pan that has been sprayed with nonstick cooking spray. Sprinkle with breadcrumbs and bake in preheated 350°F oven for about 45 minutes. Let stand 10 minutes then cut into 1-1/2 inch squares.

Per serving: 53 Calories; 2g Fat (32% calories from fat); 6g Protein; 3g Carbohydrate; 20mg Cholesterol; 158mg Sodium

Spinach Dip

Serving Size: 12

20 oz. chopped spinach, frozen
1 1/2 envelopes dry vegetable soup mix
16 oz. fat-free sour cream
1 1/2 c. reduced-fat mayonnaise
8 oz. water chestnuts, chopped
3 green onions, chopped

Cook spinach according to package directions without salt or fat. Drain. Squeeze out excess juice. Mix with remaining ingredients and refrigerate overnight.

To serve: Serve in hollowed out bread round and cube remaining bread or serve with Melba toast rounds or favorite crackers.

Per serving: 149 Calories; 9g Fat (47% calories from fat); 5g Protein; 17g Carbohydrate; 14mg Cholesterol; 310mg Sodium

Spinach Dip 2

Serving Size: 6

20 oz. frozen chopped spinach, thawed and drained
1 c. fat-free sour cream
1 c. fat-free mayonnaise
1 tsp. onion powder
1 tbsp. lemon juice
8 oz. canned water chestnuts, sliced and drained

Combine all ingredients and mix well. Refrigerate several hours. Serve with assorted fresh vegetables or fat-free crackers.

Per serving: 101 Calories; less than one gram Fat (2% calories from fat); 6g Protein; 24g Carbohydrate; 4mg Cholesterol; 609mg Sodium

Stuffed Mushrooms

Serving Size: 4

10 medium mushroom caps, cleaned
1/2 c. nonfat cottage cheese
1/2 tsp. beef broth, cubes or granules
1/2 tsp. chives, freeze-dried
1/4 tsp. Worcestershire sauce

Mix cottage cheese, bouillon granules, chives and Worcestershire sauce in blender or food processor until smooth. Stuff each cap with mixture and refrigerate until ready to serve.

Per serving: 40 Calories; less than one gram Fat (7% calories from fat); 6g Protein; 5g Carbohydrate; 1mg Cholesterol; 229mg Sodium

Tamale Balls

Serving Size: 150

1 lb. ground beef
1 lb. ground turkey
1 1/2 c. cornmeal
1/4 c. flour
3/4 c. tomato juice
3 cloves garlic, crushed
1 tbsp. chili powder
2 tsps. salt

Sauce

3 No. 2 cans tomatoes, mashed
2 tsps. salt
1 tbsp. chili powder

Blend all tamale ingredients together. Form into about 150 small balls. Set aside. Combine sauce ingredients in medium saucepan. Over medium heat, bring to a boil. Add meatballs to sauce and simmer 2 hours. Serve hot from chafing dish with toothpicks.

Per serving: 21 Calories; 1g Fat (47% calories from fat); 1g Protein; 2g Carbohydrate; 5mg Cholesterol; 67mg Sodium

The Best 7-layer Mexican Dip

Serving Size: 12

21 oz. refried beans with jalapenos
Avocado layer
3 avocados ripe
2 tbsps. lemon juice
1/2 tsp. salt
1/4 tsp. pepper
Sour cream layer
1 c. fat-free sour cream
1/2 c. reduced-fat mayonnaise
1 pkg. taco seasoning mix
Topping layer
1 bunch green onion, chopped
3 medium tomatoes, seeded and chopped
7 oz. ripe olives, chopped
8 oz. fat-free cheddar cheese, grated

Layer in order in glass casserole dish:
bean dip
avocado mixture
sour cream mixture
Sprinkle with onions, tomatoes, olives. Top with cheese. Refrigerate. Serve with corn chips.

Per serving: 220 Calories; 11g Fat (41% calories from fat); 12g Protein; 23g Carbohydrate; 9mg Cholesterol; 843mg Sodium

Tomato-Mozzarella Bites

Serving Size: 20

1 pint cherry tomatoes
1/4 lb. lowfat mozzarella cheese, diced
2 tbsps. olive oil
1 garlic clove, minced
2 tbsps. fresh basil, minced
1/4 c. sun-dried tomatoes, oil-packed and drained
black pepper

Cut mozzarella into 1/4-inch cubes. Chop fresh basil leaves finely. Mince garlic clove. Combine the cheese, basil, garlic, sun-dried tomatoes and black pepper in small bowl. Add the olive oil and blend well. Cover and refrigerate 1 hour to blend flavors. Just before serving, prepare cherry tomatoes by removing the stem end, cutting a thin slice from bottom of tomato to keep it setting straight and removing center from tomatoes with a small spoon. Sprinkle inside of tomatoes very lightly with salt and invert on paper towels to drain briefly. Stuff the tomatoes with the cheese mixture, and serve immediately.

Per serving: 34 Calories; 3g Fat (65% calories from fat); 2g Protein; 1g Carbohydrate; 3mg Cholesterol; 35mg Sodium

Tomatoes Stuffed with Salmon

Serving Size: 5

5 each roma tomatoes
6 oz. smoked salmon
1/3 c. lowfat cream cheese
1/2 tsp. Worcestershire sauce
1/3 c. green onion, chopped

Cut the tops off of each tomato then scoop out the pulp inside without damaging the whole tomato. Sprinkle the tomatoes with a little salt, and turn them upside down to drain. Meanwhile, combine salmon, cream cheese, worcestershire sauce and green onion and stir well. Spoon the salmon mixture evenly into each of the tomatoes, chill and serve.

Per serving: 101 Calories; 5g Fat (40% calories from fat); 9g Protein; 6g Carbohydrate; 16mg Cholesterol; 388mg Sodium

Tortilla Roll-Ups

Serving Size: 6

8 oz. lowfat cream cheese, softened
1/2 c. picante sauce
1 each green onion, minced
6 each flour tortillas
1 c. romaine lettuce, shredded
6 thin turkey breast slices
1/4 c. pimientos

Combine cream cheese, picante sauce, and onion. Spread evenly on each tortilla, spreading to edges. Top each with lettuce, turkey, and 2 teaspoons pimento. Roll up tightly like a jelly roll. Place seam side down in a baking dish, cover and refrigerate. Let sit at least 30 minutes to allow flavors to develop. Serve as is or with guacamole and additional picante sauce.

Per serving: 241 Calories; 10g Fat (37% calories from fat); 13g Protein; 25g Carbohydrate; 30mg Cholesterol; 882mg Sodium

Vegetable Dip with Zip

Serving Size: 4

1/4 tsp. dry mustard
3/4 c. fat-free mayonnaise
2 tbsps. chili sauce
2 tbsps. lime juice
1 tbsp. minced parsley
3 tbsps. sweet gherkins, minced
1 tsp. onion powder
1/4 tsp. Tabasco sauce, optional

Mix 2 tablespoons mayonnaise with the dry mustard. Add remaining ingredients. Mix well, refrigerate and serve with fresh cut-up vegetables.

Per serving: 55 Calories; less than one gram Fat (1% calories from fat); 0g Protein; 14g Carbohydrate; 0mg Cholesterol; 679mg Sodium

Vegetable Quesadillas

Serving Size: 12

1 1/2 c. broccoli florets, cooked and chopped
1 c. fat-free cheddar cheese, shredded
4 oz. chopped green chilies, drained
1/3 c. green onions, finely chopped
2 tbsps. cilantro, finely chopped
12 corn tortillas

Combine broccoli, cheese, green onions, chilies and cilantro in small bowl. Mix well. Cover and refrigerate until ready to use. Preheat broiler and prepare cookie sheet with nonstick cooking spray. Place 1/2 cup vegetable filling on half of tortilla. Fold over other side to enclose filling and into a turnover. Broil 1 1/2 to 2 1/2 minutes on each side. Cut into wedges to serve.

Per serving: 79 Calories; 1g Fat (8% calories from fat); 5g Protein; 14g Carbohydrate; 2mg Cholesterol; 112mg Sodium

Breads

Buttermilk Whole Wheat Bread

Serving Size: 10

1 c. all-purpose flour
1 c. whole wheat flour
1/2 tsp. salt
1/2 tsp. baking soda
1/2 tsp. sugar
1 tbsp. canola oil
1 c. low-fat buttermilk
1 egg, beaten

Sift all dry ingredients together. Add oil and 3/4 cup of buttermilk and stir to make a soft dough, adding more buttermilk if needed. Shape dough into a round loaf and brush with beaten egg. Place in an oven that has been preheated to 400°F and bake for 30 minutes.

Per serving: 115 Calories; 2g Fat (18% calories from fat); 4g Protein; 20g Carbohydrate; 19mg Cholesterol; 201mg Sodium

Fat-Free French Bread

Serving Size: 8

2 1/2 tsps. dry yeast
3 c. bread flour
1/2 tsp. salt
1 1/2 tsps. sugar
1 1/2 cups water

Place all ingredients in bread maker. Set for French bread cycle on medium brown crust.

Per serving: 192 Calories; 1g Fat (4% calories from fat); 7g Protein; 39g Carbohydrate; 0mg Cholesterol; 136mg Sodium

Focaccia

Serving Size: 10

1 tbsp. dry yeast (one pkg.)
1 pinch sugar
2 c. warm water, 110°F
1 tbsp. minced garlic
1 tsp. chopped fresh rosemary
1 tsp. chopped fresh oregano
extra virgin olive oil
kosher salt (if available)

4 1/2 c. bread flour
1 1/4 tsps. salt
1/4 c. extra virgin olive oil
1 tsp. chopped fresh basil
1 tbsp. minced shallots
coarsely ground pepper

In a large bowl, place the yeast in the bottom and slowly add the water and pinch of sugar. Let yeast sit for 5 minutes, then stir to dissolve the yeast. Combine the salt and flour, set aside. Add the olive oil, garlic, shallots and herbs to the water mixture. Stir in the flour mixture with a heavy spoon, eventually switching to your hands to incorporate all the flour. Knead the dough for 10 minutes until the dough is very elastic. Place the dough in a bowl that has been lightly oiled with some of the olive oil, and rub a little extra on top of the dough. Cover the bowl with plastic and set aside in a warm place to rise until doubled in size, about 1-1 1/2 hours. Take dough out of bowl and knead the dough again for about 2 minutes, or until the air has all been pushed out of the dough. Gently stretch out the dough into a 11 X 17 inch baking sheet that has been sprayed with nonstick cooking spray, making sure the dough is of even thickness on every side. Pour about a tablespoon of olive oil on top of the bread and rub it all over the top of the dough. Lightly sprinkle the dough with kosher salt and pepper and let the bread sit at room temperature for 30 minutes.

Preheat oven to 400°F. Place bread in the oven and bake for 15 minutes. Reduce heat to 350°F and continue to bake for 20 minutes more, or until crust is golden. Remove pan from oven and allow bread to cool 5 minutes before cutting or removing the bread from the pan.

Notes: Focaccia can be made with any variety of herbs and spices that you like. Another good recipe uses sage and thyme instead of basil, rosemary and oregano. Also, the amount of herbs used can be increased or decreased, depending on your taste.

Per serving: 276 Calories; 6g Fat (21% calories from fat); 8g Protein; 46g Carbohydrate; 0mg Cholesterol; 270mg Sodium

Garlic Bread

Serving Size: 6

1 pound French bread
1/2 c. fat-free mayonnaise
1/4 c. fat-free Parmesan cheese
1 1/2 tsps. minced garlic

Combine mayonnaise, cheese and garlic in small bowl. Mix well. Slice bread in half lengthwise and spread both side with mixture. Place on cookie sheet and bake at 450°F for 10 minutes or until heated thoroughly.

Per serving: 236 Calories; 2g Fat (9% calories from fat); 8g Protein; 45g Carbohydrate; 4mg Cholesterol; 750mg Sodium

Nutty Wheat Bread

Serving Size: 10

1 1/4 c. warm water
2 tsps. yeast
1/4 c. maltitol, honey flavored
1/2 tsp. salt
1 1/2 c. bread flour
1 1/2 c. whole wheat flour
3 tbsps. wheat germ
3/4 c. chopped almonds toasted

In a large bowl, place the yeast in the bottom and slowly add the water and maltitol. Let yeast sit for 5 minutes, then stir to dissolve the yeast. Combine the remaining ingredients. Stir in the flour mixture with a heavy spoon, eventually switching to your hands to incorporate all the flour. Knead the dough for 10 minutes until the dough is very elastic. Place the dough in a bowl that has been lightly oiled, and rub a little extra on top of the dough. Cover the bowl with plastic and set aside in a warm place to rise until doubled in size, about 1-1 1/2 hours. Take dough out of bowl and knead the dough again for about 2 minutes, or until the air has all been pushed out of the dough. Roll the dough into a 8 X 10 rectangle and roll it up to be a 8 inch long loaf. Place in a bread loaf pan that has been sprayed with nonstick cooking spray and let rise until the dough just peeks over the edge of the pan. Place the bread in an oven that has been preheated to 375°F and bake for 30 - 35 minutes, or until bread is golden brown. Let bread cool in pan before removing, then take out the loaf and let it lay on its side until it is completely cool.

Per serving: 223 Calories; 7g Fat (25% calories from fat); 8g Protein; 36g Carbohydrate; 0mg Cholesterol; 111mg Sodium

Peach Perfect Muffins

Serving Size: 12

1 c. whole wheat flour
1 c. oat bran
1 tbsp. baking powder
1/4 c. maltitol, plus 2 tbsps.
1/4 c. plain low-fat yogurt, plus 2 tbsps.
3 tbsps. prunes, pureed
2 egg whites
1 tsp. vanilla
1 c. fresh peaches, chopped
1/3 c. raisins

Mix dry ingredients. Add the maltitol, yogurt, prune puree, egg whites and vanilla. Stir until moist. Fold in peaches and the raisins. Prepare muffin cups with nonstick cooking spray. Fill cups 3/4 full. Bake at 350°F for 15 to 17 minutes or until done. Cool 5 minutes before removing from pan. Serve warm or room temperature.

Per serving: 94 Calories; 1g Fat (7% calories from fat); 4g Protein; 23g Carbohydrate; 0mg Cholesterol; 105mg Sodium

Pita Pizzas

Serving Size: 4

4 pita bread rounds
2 tsps. olive oil
1/4 c. chopped onion
2 cloves garlic, minced
1/2 c. pizza sauce
2 tsps. dried basil
1 large green bell pepper
1 c. low-fat mozzarella cheese, shredded

Preheat oven to 425°F. Bake each pita for 5 minutes or until crisp. Heat oil in a small saucepan over medium heat then add onion. Cook onion for about 7 minutes or until it is soft. Add garlic and cook 1 minute more. Combine pizza sauce and basil and spread on pitas. Top with onion mixture, bell pepper and mozzarella cheese then bake for 5-7 minutes or until cheese is melted.

Per serving: 297 Calories; 9g Fat (27% calories from fat); 14g Protein; 40g Carbohydrate; 15mg Cholesterol; 669mg Sodium

Pretzels

Serving Size: 12

1 envelope active dry yeast
3/4 c. warm water (105°-115°F)
2 1/2 c. whole wheat flour
1 large egg white

Combine yeast and warm water in large bowl. Let stand 5 minutes. Stir until yeast dissolves. Add 1 1/2 cups flour; beat with spoon until smooth. Turn dough onto lightly floured surface and knead 5 minutes. Spray large bowl lightly with nonstick cooking spray. Shape dough into ball and place in bowl, turning several times. Cover with clean dish towel and place in warm spot until dough doubles in size, approximately 1 1/2 hours.

Punch dough down and divide in half. Cut each half into 6 pieces. Roll each piece into 18 inch long pieces. Twist into pretzel shapes. Tuck ends under. Place pretzels on cookie sheet that has been prepared with nonstick cooking spray approximately 1 inch apart. Cover with towel. Let pretzels rise in warm spot 30 minutes. Brush pretzels with egg white that has been beaten with 1 teaspoon water and bake at 400°F for 10 to 15 minutes or until golden brown.

Notes: This recipe can be used to make bread sticks. Follow recipe and instead of shaping into pretzels, leave in 18 inch strips. Bake 20 minutes at 350°F. Garlic or onion powder can be added to dough for flavor.

Per serving: 89 Calories; 1g Fat (5% calories from fat); 4g Protein; 19g Carbohydrate; 0mg Cholesterol; 7mg Sodium

Strawberry Oatmeal Muffins

Serving Size: 12

1 1/4 c. quick-cooking oats
1 1/4 c. buttermilk
1 1/4 c. whole wheat flour
1/3 c. maltitol
1 tbsp. baking powder
1/4 tsp. baking soda
3 tbsps. prunes, pureed
2 egg whites
1 tsp. vanilla
1 c. strawberries, chopped

Combine oats and buttermilk and set aside for at least 5 minutes. Combine the next 4 ingredients; add oat/buttermilk mixture, prune puree, egg whites and vanilla. Stir just until dry ingredients are moist. Fold in strawberries. Fill muffin cups that have been prepared with nonstick cooking spray 3/4 full. Bake at 350°F for 15 to 17 minutes or until done. Cool for 15 minutes before removing from pan. Serve warm or at room temperature.

Per serving: 114 Calories; 1g Fat (8% calories from fat); 5g Protein; 24g Carbohydrate; 1mg Cholesterol; 154mg Sodium

Sugar Free Sticky Buns

Serving Size: 8

1/2 c. maltitol-sweetened butterscotch sauce
1/4 tsp. cinnamon
1/4 c. raisins, optional
1/4 c. pecans, optional
1 pkg. low-fat biscuit dough

Prepare 8 or 9 inch square baking pan with nonstick cooking spray. Add ingredients in order given, ending with biscuits. Bake at 450°F for 10 minutes then at 400°F for 4 minutes. Remove from oven and invert.

Per serving: 70 Calories; 1g Fat (16% calories from fat); 1g Protein; 17g Carbohydrate; 0mg Cholesterol; 76mg Sodium

Vegetable Pizza Crust

Serving Size: 8

3/4 c. zucchini, grated or 3/4 c. yellow squash, grated
1/2 c. carrot, grated
1/2 c. red and green bell peppers, minced
2 tsps. salt
2 each eggs
1/2 c. mozzarella cheese, grated
1/2 c. Parmesan cheese, grated

Combine zucchini or squash with carrot and bell peppers in a colander and sprinkle salt over them. Mix in the salt a little, then allow the vegetables to drain for 15 minutes. Rinse the vegetables afterwards and squeeze all excess water out of them. Combine drained vegetables in a large bowl with the eggs and cheeses. Preheat the oven to 375°F and spray a meduim sized pizza pan with nonstick cooking spray. Press the mtixture evenly into the pan, then bake until crisp, about 15 minutes.

Per serving: 72 Calories; 4g Fat (54% calories from fat); 5g Protein; 3g Carbohydrate; 56mg Cholesterol; 674mg Sodium

Soups and Stews

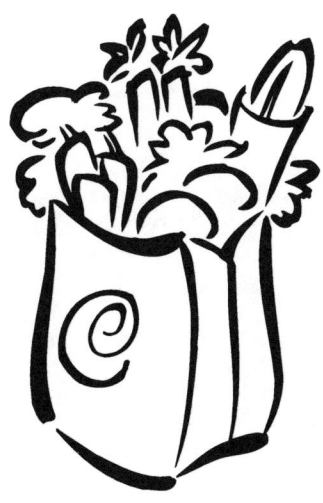

Bean and Cabbage Soup

Serving Size: 6

4 c. fat-free beef broth
1 c. water
1 medium cabbage, coarsely chopped
1 1/2 c. carrots, sliced
1 c. onion, sliced
1/2 tsp. ground allspice
19 oz. canned white beans, rinsed and drained
2 tbsps. dried dill
fat-free sour cream, optional

Combine all ingredients except beans, dill and sour cream in large soup pot. Bring to boil. Reduce heat. Cover. Simmer 15 minutes or until vegetables are crisp-tender. Add beans and dill. Simmer, uncovered 5 minutes. Garnish with sour cream, if desired.

Per serving: 162 Calories; 1g Fat (3% calories from fat); 16g Protein; 31g Carbohydrate; 0mg Cholesterol; 784mg Sodium

Bean and Pasta Stew

Serving Size: 4

1 c. tomato, coarsely chopped
3/4 c. shell pasta, uncooked
1/4 c. onion, chopped
1/4 c. green bell pepper, chopped
1 tsp. dried basil
3 cloves garlic, minced
16 oz. kidney beans, canned and drained
14 1/2 oz. chicken broth, canned
8 oz. white beans, canned and drained
1/4 c. grated Parmesan cheese

Mix all ingredients, except Parmesan cheese, in a 2 quart saucepan. Heat until boiling, stirring occasionally. Reduce heat to a simmer, cover and simmer until pasta is tender. Garnish each serving with Parmesan cheese.

Per serving: 285 Calories; 4g Fat (12% calories from fat); 16g Protein; 47g Carbohydrate; 6mg Cholesterol; 1410mg Sodium

Black Bean Chili

Serving Size: 6

1 large onion, chopped
2 red bell peppers, seeded and chopped
1 tbsp. chopped jalapeno
10 mushrooms, quartered
6 small tomatoes, cut in quarters
1 c. frozen corn kernels, thawed and drained
1 tsp. pepper
1 tsp. ground cumin
1 tbsp. chili powder
4 c. black beans, cooked and rinsed
1 1/2 c. fat-free chicken broth
10 oz. frozen chopped spinach, thawed and drained

Add onion, red pepper, jalapeno, mushrooms, tomatoes, corn, pepper, cumin and chili powder to skillet that has been prepared with nonstick cooking spray. Cook over medium heat for 10 minutes, stirring constantly. Add beans and chicken broth. Bring to boil and boil 10 minutes. Remove 1 1/2 cup bean mixture from skillet and place in blender or food processor. Blend until pureed. Return to saucepan and add spinach. Cook 5 to 6 minutes more or until spinach is heated thoroughly.

Per serving: 258 Calories; 2g Fat (6% calories from fat); 18g Protein; 50g Carbohydrate; 0mg Cholesterol; 195mg Sodium

Chicken Corn Chowder

Serving Size: 6

10 3/4 oz. cream of celery soup, condensed
10 3/4 oz. skim milk
1/2 c. salsa
8 oz. corn, canned and drained
1 c. cooked chicken breast halves, cubed
4 slices Canadian bacon, chopped
1/2 c. nonfat cheddar cheese
1 tbsp. minced fresh chives

Combine all ingredients except cheese and chives in a 2 quart sauce pot over medium heat until simmering. Remove from heat, garnish each bowl with cheese and chives before serving.

Per serving: 190 Calories; 7g Fat (31% calories from fat); 20g Protein; 14g Carbohydrate; 44mg Cholesterol; 1008mg Sodium

Chicken-flavored Vegetable Soup

Serving Size: 8

8 cans fat-free chicken broth
6 carrots, peeled and cubed
6 stalks celery, cut in large pieces
16 oz. broccoli florets
16 oz. cauliflower florets
16 oz. green beans

In large soup pot, bring chicken broth to boil. Add carrots and celery. Cook over medium heat, 20 minutes or until tender. Add broccoli, cauliflower and green beans. Continue to cook 10 to 20 minutes.

Fat-free noodles or matzo balls can be added. Add noodles in the last 10 minutes of cooking time.

Per serving: 93 Calories; 1g Fat (3% calories from fat); 18g Protein; 18g Carbohydrate; 0mg Cholesterol; 702mg Sodium

Cream of Onion Soup

Serving Size: 6

6 c. sliced onion
1/4 c. reduced-calorie margarine
dash ground nutmeg
3 tbsps. flour
2 c. milk
1 c. chicken broth
Salt to taste
Parmesan cheese, grated
1 1/2 c. croutons

Over medium heat, saute onions in margarine until deep gold. Sprinkle with nutmeg and flour, and stir until a paste forms. Add milk slowly, stirring constantly until slightly thickened. Add chicken broth. Bring to a simmer, reduce heat and cook 20 minutes. Serve with cheese and croutons.

Per serving: 196 Calories; 8g Fat (35% calories from fat); 6g Protein; 27g Carbohydrate; 11mg Cholesterol; 451mg Sodium

Cream of Vegetable Soup

Serving Size: 6

2 c. fat-free chicken broth
20 oz. frozen mixed vegetables
1 c. cooked rice
2 c. skim milk
pepper to taste
1/2 tsp. onion powder
1/2 tsp. garlic powder

Combine chicken broth and vegetables in large saucepan. Bring to boil over high heat. Reduce heat to low, cover. Simmer until vegetables are tender, stirring occasionally. Pour half the broth, half of the vegetables and the cooked rice into blender and blend at low speed until smooth. Pour into large bowl, repeat with rest of broth and vegetables. Stir milk and spices into soup mixture. Heat thoroughly. Soup may be served hot or cold.

Per serving: 137 Calories; 1g Fat (4% calories from fat); 11g Protein; 26g Carbohydrate; 1mg Cholesterol; 260mg Sodium

Easy Gazpacho

Serving Size: 8

4 large chopped tomatoes, without seeds
1 each bell pepper, chopped
1 each cucumber
1 c. chopped celery
4 c. tomato juice
3 tbsps. red wine vinegar
1/2 tsp. black pepper
2 tbsps. fresh lemon juice

Peel cucumber and cut in half lengthwise. Scoop out seeds with a teaspoon, then chop. Combine cucumber with all other ingredients in a large glass or plastic container and refrigerate overnight before serving.

Per serving: 62 Calories; 1g Fat (7% calories from fat); 3g Protein; 15g Carbohydrate; 0mg Cholesterol; 466mg Sodium

Fat-Free Matzo Balls

Serving Size: 10

4 egg whites
1/2 c. matzo meal
2 tsps. dried onions
1/2 tsp. cinnamon
1 tsp. dried parsley
1/4 tsp. pepper

Beat egg whites in large bowl until stiff. In separate bowl, combine matzo meal and spices. Fold into egg whites. Let stand 15 minutes. Form mixture into small balls with your hands. To keep dough from sticking to your hands, spray lightly with nonstick cooking spray or water. Drop matzo balls into boiling water or soup. Cover pot and simmer 30 minutes. Matzo balls can be frozen and added to soup when ready to serve.

Per serving: 34 Calories; less than one gram Fat (3% calories from fat); 2g Protein; 6g Carbohydrate; 0mg Cholesterol; 22mg Sodium

French Onion Soup

Serving Size: 12

5 lbs. yellow onions, sliced thin
6 oz. fat-free margarine
21 oz. nonfat beef broth, canned or fresh
3/4 c. flour
paprika to taste
pepper to taste
12 slices sourdough bread
1/3 c. fat-free Swiss cheese

Melt margarine in large soup pot. Add onion slices and simmer over low heat 2 hours. Drain liquid from pot, leaving enough to coat onions. Add flour, paprika and pepper. Cook about 10 minutes or until the onion mixture thickens. Add the broth. Cover, cook over low heat 1 1/2 hours. Bake the bread slices at 350°F for 10 minutes on each side. To serve, place on slice of bread in each oven proof soup bowl and cover with soup. Top with cheese. Place bowls under broiler and cook until cheese is melted.

Serving Ideas: Best if soup is prepared a day ahead and refrigerated.

Per serving: 187 Calories; 1g Fat (7% calories from fat); 6g Protein; 38g Carbohydrate; 1mg Cholesterol; 405mg Sodium

Gazpacho Soup

Serving Size: 8

3 large cans stewed tomatoes, Mexican-style
3 stalks celery
1 green pepper
1 red pepper
4 oz. chopped green chilies
1 cucumber
2 tbsps. Worcestershire sauce
1 tsp. garlic powder
1 tsp. onion powder
pepper to taste

Place stewed tomatoes in large bowl. Chop all vegetables into chunky pieces. Add to tomatoes. Add remaining ingredients. Chill before serving. Keeps well in refrigerator for several days.

Per serving: 55 Calories; 1g Fat (18% calories from fat); 2g Protein; 11g Carbohydrate; 0mg Cholesterol; 223mg Sodium

Ham and Lima Bean Stew

Serving Size: 8

3 ham hocks, smoked	1 lb. lima beans
3 c. nonfat chicken broth	3 c. water
2 garlic cloves	2 sweet onions
1 c. celery, diced	1 c. carrots, sliced
hot pepper sauce, optional	1 bay leaf

Prepare lima beans by picking over to remove any debris that might be in package. Rinse beans well. Cover with about 8 cups water. Bring to a boil, cover and boil 2 minutes. Remove from heat, keep covered and allow to stand for 1 hour or more. While beans are soaking, prepare the ham hocks (or use meaty ham bones). Combine the 3 cups broth and 3 cups water in a large heavy pan with lid; bring to a boil. Add the ham and simmer for about 1 hour. Drain the beans, running hot water over beans briefly to rinse. Add the beans to the ham mixture. Slice the onions and separate into rings. Add the onions, along with the carrots, celery, and bay leaf, to the pot. Mince the garlic cloves; add to mixture. Ham is salted already so you may not want to add salt at this point. Pour additional broth or hot water over this mixture to reach about 1 inch above the ingredients. Simmer for about 1 hour, stirring several times, checking to see if you need to add more liquid. After beans and vegetables are tender, remove the ham hocks or bone. Remove the meat from bones and add back to the bean mixture. Taste and add more salt or pepper if you wish; also add hot pepper sauce to your taste.

Per serving: 316 Calories; 8g Fat (21% calories from fat); 23g Protein; 41g Carbohydrate; 38mg Cholesterol; 185mg Sodium

Hamburger Soup

Serving Size: 6

1 lb. extra lean ground beef
1 large can tomato juice, low sodium
Tomato juice can of water
1 large onion, chopped
3 ribs celery, chopped
2 c. cabbage, shredded
2 turnips, chopped
Parsley
Salt
Pepper
1 large bag frozen mixed vegetables
16 oz. creamed corn, low calorie
Cooked Spaghetti, optional

Saute ground beef until it looses its red color. Add tomato juice and water. Add chopped raw vegetables and simmer. Add frozen mixed vegetables and creamed corn. Simmer for several hours until heated thoroughly and vegetables are tender. Add the spaghetti, if desired. Add salt and pepper to taste, and garnish each bowl with a little chopped parsley

Per serving: 283 Calories; 14g Fat (42% calories from fat); 18g Protein; 25g Carbohydrate; 52mg Cholesterol; 114mg Sodium

Melon Soup for Summer

Serving Size: 6

3 c. cantaloupe
3 c. honeydew melon
1/4 c. lime juice
1 tsp. honey
1/4 c. plain nonfat yogurt

Peel, seed, and chop each melon. Place chopped melon in a blender and add remaining ingredients to blender. Blend until completely smooth. Serve cold, with a swirl of yogurt in the middle.

Per serving: 40 Calories; less than one gram Fat (4% calories from fat); 1g Protein; 10g Carbohydrate; 0mg Cholesterol; 15mg Sodium

Mushroom Barley Soup

Serving Size: 4

2 yellow onion, chopped
3 carrots, peeled and sliced
1/2 lb. mushrooms, sliced
4 c. fat-free beef broth
1/4 c. chopped parsley
1/2 c. barley
 pepper to taste

Combine all ingredients in large pot and bring to boil. Lower heat so soup boils gently. Simmer, partly covered, 40 minutes or until barley is tender.

Per serving: 152 Calories; 1g Fat (4% calories from fat); 16g Protein; 30g Carbohydrate; 0mg Cholesterol; 543mg Sodium

Potato Chowder

Serving Size: 4

2 tbsps. reduced-calorie margarine
2 c. potatoes, diced and uncooked
2 green onion, chopped
1 clove garlic, chopped
1 can chicken noodle soup
14 1/2 oz. canned tomatoes, peeled
1/4 tsp. black pepper, optional
1 c. skim milk

Place margarine and potatoes in nonstick pot. Cook, stirring constantly until potatoes are transparent. Add green onions, garlic and chicken noodle soup. Chop tomatoes and add with juice. Add pepper if desired. Cover and simmer until potatoes are tender, approximately 25 minutes. Add milk. Continue to cook until thoroughly heated. Serve immediately.

Per serving: 181 Calories; 4g Fat (19% calories from fat); 7g Protein; 32g Carbohydrate; 3mg Cholesterol; 562mg Sodium

Southwestern Black Bean Soup

Serving Size: 8

2 tsps. canola oil
1 medium onion, chopped
3 cloves garlic, minced
1 tsp. dried oregano
1/2 tsp. dried thyme
1 tsp. cumin powder
1 dash cayenne pepper
3 c. cooked black beans, rinsed and drained
3 c. chicken broth
1/4 c. fresh cilantro, chopped
2 tomatoes, chopped
1/2 c. low-fat sour cream, optional

Heat oil in a 3 or 4 quart saucepan over medium heat. Add onion and saute until tender. While onions are cooking, place half the beans in a blender with some of the broth and blend until completely smooth, set aside. Once onion is soft, add garlic and spices, and cook one minute more. Add pureed beans, whole beans and remaining broth to sauce pot, and bring to a boil. Lower heat and simmer uncovered for 20-30 minutes. Stir in cilantro just before serving and garnish with tomatoes and sour cream.

Per serving: 148 Calories; 3g Fat (20% calories from fat); 8g Protein; 22g Carbohydrate; 4mg Cholesterol; 609mg Sodium

Tortilla Soup

Serving Size: 8

1 small onion, chopped
4 oz. green chilies, chopped
2 cloves garlic, chopped
2 tbsps. oil
1 tsp. cumin
1 tsp. salt
1 tsp. chili powder
1/8 tsp. coarsely ground pepper
2 tsps. Worcestershire sauce
1 tsp. bottled steak sauce
1 c. tomatoes, peeled and chopped
1 can chicken broth
1 can beef broth
1 1/2 c. water
3 corn tortillas cut in 1/2" strips
1/4 c. Monterey Jack cheese, grated
1/4 c. cilantro, chopped

In large pot, saute onion, green chilies and garlic in oil. Add remaining ingredients except tortillas, cheese and cilantro. Simmer, covered for 1 hour. Add cilantro; cook 10 minutes more. Garnish with tortilla strips and grated cheese.
Notes: Great made a day ahead and reheated.

Per serving: 94 Calories; 6g Fat (54% calories from fat); 3g Protein; 9g Carbohydrate; 4mg Cholesterol; 807mg Sodium

Tuna Chowder

Serving Size: 8

8 mushrooms, sliced
2 stalks celery, diagonally sliced
1 medium onion, diced
1 large potato, diced
4 c. fat-free chicken broth
12 oz. evaporated skim milk
24 oz. tuna in water, do not drain
 salt and pepper to taste

Combine mushrooms, celery, onion, potato and chicken broth in large pot. Add evaporated milk and tuna. Bring to boil. Reduce heat and cover. Simmer 30 minutes, stirring occasionally. Season to taste with salt and pepper before serving.

Per serving: 180 Calories; 1g Fat (4% calories from fat); 32g Protein; 15g Carbohydrate; 27mg Cholesterol; 606mg Sodium

Vegetable Soup

Serving Size: 8

3 1/4 c. fat-free chicken broth, divided
1 1/4 lb.s yams, peeled and cubed
3 carrots, peeled and cubed
1 1/2 c. onions, diced
8 oz. mushrooms, sliced
2 cloves garlic, minced
1 tsp. Italian seasoning
1/2 tsp. pepper
5 c. water
3/4 c. pasta shells, small
10 oz. frozen peas
10 oz. spinach leaves, fresh or frozen

Heat 2 to 3 tablespoons chicken broth in large soup pot over medium high heat. Add yams, carrots, onions, mushrooms, garlic, Italian seasoning and pepper. Cook, stirring constantly, until vegetables begin to brown. Add remaining chicken broth and water to pot. Bring to boil. Reduce heat to low, cover, simmer 20 minutes. Bring to boil again. Over medium-high heat, add pasta. Cook, uncovered 5 minutes. Add peas and spinach. Return to boil. Cook until pasta is tender, approximately 5 minutes.

Per serving: 179 Calories; 1g Fat (3% calories from fat); 10g Protein; 38g Carbohydrate; 0mg Cholesterol; 292mg Sodium

Vegetarian Chili

Serving Size: 8

1 c. chopped onion
1/2 c. green bell pepper, chopped
2 tbsps. canola oil
4 cloves garlic, minced
2 c. chopped zucchini
1 c. chopped carrots
32 oz. canned pinto beans, rinsed and drained
32 oz. canned tomatoes, diced, with juice
2 tbsps. chili powder
1 tsp. cumin
1/2 tsp. dried oregano
1/2 tsp. black pepper
1/2 c. water

In a 3 or 4 quart sauce pot, saute onion and green bell pepper in canola oil over medium heat until onions are soft. Add garlic, zucchini and carrot and cook for 2 minutes more. Add beans, tomatoes, spices and water and stir to combine everything. Bring to a boil, reduce heat and simmer for about a half hour, or until vegetables are tender. Serve garnished with cheddar cheese, if desired.

Per serving: 169 Calories; 5g Fat (23% calories from fat); 7g Protein; 27g Carbohydrate; 0mg Cholesterol; 739mg Sodium

Yogurt Soup for a Hot Day

Serving Size: 4

1 cucumber, peeled and sliced
1 tomato peeled, seeded
3 tbsps. sweet onions, chopped
2 tbsps. fresh mint, chopped
1 c. nonfat plain yogurt
6 mint sprigs
1 dash cayenne pepper

Put the cucumber, tomato, onion and mint into a food processor or blender. Process until smooth. Add the yogurt and blend well. To make by hand, chop the cucumber, onion and mint finely, reserving as much liquid as possible. Put the chopped ingredients and any reserved liquid into a mixing bowl and add the remaining ingredients. Serve chilled, garnished with a sprig of mint and a sprinkling of cayenne pepper.

Per serving: 54 Calories; less than one gram Fat (5% calories from fat); 4g Protein; 9g Carbohydrate; 1mg Cholesterol; 47mg Sodium

Salads and Salad Dressings

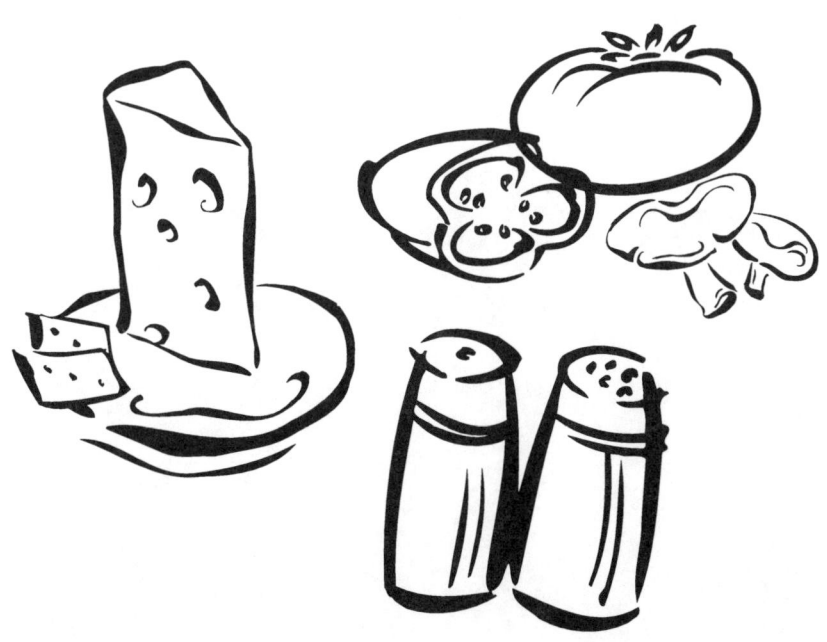

Cheddar Pea Salad

Serving Size: 6

16 oz. English peas, drained
1 c. lowfat cheddar cheese, grated
1/2 c. chopped celery
1 hard-boiled egg, chopped
1 tbsp. grated onion, optional
1/4 c. reduced-calorie mayonnaise

Combine all ingredients. Mix well. Cover and refrigerate at least 1 hour before serving.

Per serving: 156 Calories; 7g Fat (40% calories from fat); 11g Protein; 13g Carbohydrate; 43mg Cholesterol; 184mg Sodium

Chicken Salad

Serving Size: 6

8 each chicken breasts without skin, cooked and cubed
1 c. celery, chopped fine
1/2 tsp. garlic powder, coarsely ground
  with parsley
1/2 c. reduced-calorie mayonnaise
1/3 c. low-fat mayonnaise
1 medium Red Delicious apple, shredded

In large bowl, combine all ingredients except apple. Mix well. Sprinkle with apple. Toss. If salad is too dry, add a little more mayonnaise.

Per serving: 433 Calories; 13g Fat (28% calories from fat); 69g Protein; 6g Carbohydrate; 184mg Cholesterol; 367mg Sodium

Corn and Bean Salad

Serving Size: 10

30 oz. canned kidney beans, rinsed and drained
1 1/2 c. corn
1/2 c. chopped green onions, tops included
1/2 c. bell pepper, chopped
1/3 c. white wine vinegar
1/3 c. water
1/8 tsp. cayenne pepper
1 tsp. celery seed

In a medium bowl, combine beans, corn, onion and bell pepper, set aside. In a small saucepan, bring vinegar, water and cayenne pepper to a boil and cook one minute. Remove from heat and stir in celery seed. Pour over vegetable mixture and toss. Cover and refrigerate for at least 8 hours before serving, stirring every now and then.

Per serving: 98 Calories; 1g Fat (6% calories from fat); 5g Protein; 19g Carbohydrate; 0mg Cholesterol; 295mg Sodium

Crab or Shrimp Salad

Serving Size: 8

Salad Mix
1 c. celery
1 c. white onions
1/2 c. bell pepper
4 hard-boiled eggs
2/3 c. reduced-calorie mayonnaise
1 c. remoulade sauce
2 1/2 tsps. salt
1 tsp. black pepper
3 oz. lump crabmeat or 4 oz. shrimp, cut in half

To make salad mix: Chop celery, onions and bell peppers. Break eggs into medium-sized pieces.
To make salads:
For Crab Salad
    Mix crabmeat and Salad mix. Chill well.
For Shrimp Salad:
    Mix shrimp and Salad mix. Chill well.
To serve: Place on sliced tomatoes or bed of lettuce.

Per serving: 164 Calories; 12g Fat (60% calories from fat); 9g Protein; 9g Carbohydrate; 127mg Cholesterol; 851mg Sodium

Dill Salmon Salad

Serving Size: 4

14 oz. canned salmon, drained and flaked
1 tbsp. fresh lemon juice
2 tbsps. fresh dill, chopped
4 oz. nonfat sour cream
8 cherry tomatoes
1 head Boston lettuce, washed and torn

Combine salmon, lemon juice, dill, sour cream and tomatoes, and stir until everything is combined. Place lettuce evenly on 4 plates and portion out salmon mixture on top of the lettuce. Garnish with additional dill sprigs, if desired.

Per serving: 242 Calories; 7g Fat (26% calories from fat); 26g Protein; 22g Carbohydrate; 59mg Cholesterol; 605mg Sodium

German Cucumber Salad

Serving Size: 4

2 large cucumbers
4 oz. lowfat sour cream
2 tsps. fresh dill, chopped
1 small onion, sliced very thin
1 tsp. white wine vinegar

Peel cucumbers and cut them in half lengthwise. Scoop out the seeds with a teaspoon and slice the cucumbers very thin. Place the cucumbers in a colander and sprinkle them with about a tablespoon of salt. Let the cucumbers drain for about a half hour and rinse them. Squeeze out any excess liquid. Toss the cucumbers with the remaining ingredients and chill until cucumbers are cold.

Per serving: 86 Calories; 2g Fat (18% calories from fat); 4g Protein; 15g Carbohydrate; 6mg Cholesterol; 39mg Sodium

Grape Salad

Serving Size: 6

4 c. seedless grapes, whole
8 oz. lowfat sour cream
4 tbsps. brown sugar replacement
3/4 c. pecans, toasted and chopped

Wash grapes. Cut 2 cups of grapes in half. Mix sour cream, brown sugar replacement and pecans. Add to grapes. Refrigerate overnight. Mix well before serving.

Per serving: 158 Calories; 7g Fat (37% calories from fat); 3g Protein; 23g Carbohydrate; 8mg Cholesterol; 53mg Sodium

Green Bean Salad

Serving Size: 8

2 cans green beans, drained
1/4 c. chopped onion
1/3 c. salad oil
1/4 c. wine vinegar
1 tsp. salt
1 tsp. pepper
1/4 c. Parmesan cheese

Wash green beans. Drain. Put beans in flat dish and sprinkle with onions. In small bowl, combine oil, vinegar, salt and pepper. Pour over beans and onions. Sprinkle with Parmesan cheese. Cover and marinate overnight.

Per serving: 103 Calories; 10g Fat (83% calories from fat); 2g Protein; 3g Carbohydrate; 2mg Cholesterol; 315mg Sodium

Green Pea and Blue Cheese Salad

Serving Size: 5

20 oz. frozen green peas, blanched
2 green onion, finely chopped
1 can pimiento, chopped
1 c. diced celery
8 oz. canned water chestnuts, drained and sliced

Marinade

1/2 c. fat-free blue cheese salad dressing
1/2 tsp. pepper
1 oz. blue cheese

Combine salad ingredients in large bowl. Add marinade ingredients. Marinate 6 hours or overnight in refrigerator before serving.

Per serving: 196 Calories; 2g Fat (10% calories from fat); 10g Protein; 37g Carbohydrate; 4mg Cholesterol; 532mg Sodium

Green Pea and Rice Salad

Serving Size: 6

1 tbsp. vinegar
2/3 c. reduced-calorie mayonnaise
1 tsp. salt
1 tsp. curry powder, optional
1/2 c. uncooked rice
2 tbsps. chopped onion
1 c. chopped celery
1 pkg. frozen peas, cooked

Mix vinegar, oil, mayonnaise, salt and curry powder. Cook rice until done according to package directions without adding salt or fat. Add rice to dressing mixture. While rice is still hot, add onions. Cool to room temperature. Add celery and peas. Refrigerate.

Per serving: 142 Calories; 7g Fat (47% calories from fat); 2g Protein; 17g Carbohydrate; 9mg Cholesterol; 513mg Sodium

Jicama and Citrus Salad

Serving Size: 6

2 c. jicama, peeled and julienned
1 large red bell pepper, sliced into rings
1 c. orange sections
1 c. grapefruit sections
1 tbsp. chopped fresh mint
1/2 c. fresh squeezed orange juice
1 tbsp. lemon juice

Combine all ingredients and serve alone or on a bed of lettuce.

Per serving: 56 Calories; less than one gram Fat (3% calories from fat); 1g Protein; 14g Carbohydrate; 0mg Cholesterol; 2mg Sodium

Corn Relish

Serving Size: 8

16 oz. low sodium canned corn, drained
or 16 oz. low sodium frozen corn, thawed
1/2 c. parsley, chopped
1 bunch green onions, chopped
1 green pepper, chopped
1 red pepper, chopped
7 1/2 oz. hearts of palm, rinsed and drained
20 cherry tomatoes, halved
4 tbsps. white wine vinegar with herbs
1 tsp. dried tarragon, crushed
1 tsp. dry mustard

Drain corn and reserve liquid. Cut heart of palm into 1/4 inch circles and combine with corn, parsley, green onions, green and red peppers and tomatoes.

To make dressing: Combine rest of ingredients and 1/2 cup of the corn liquid. Blend well. Toss vegetable mixture with dressing and marinate 2 to 4 hours before serving.

Per serving: 171 Calories; 2g Fat (9% calories from fat); 7g Protein; 40g Carbohydrate; 0mg Cholesterol; 60mg Sodium

Quick Pasta Salad

Serving Size: 6

12 oz. pasta, multicolored
1 bottle low calorie Italian salad dressing
  Any vegetables desired

Cook pasta according to package directions without salt or fat. Rinse with cool water. Add salad dressing and vegetables or leave plain. Refrigerate.

Notes: Vegetables such as broccoli, asparagus, cauliflower, carrots or even olives are great in pasta salad. For an even quicker salad, try using a bag of frozen vegetables instead of fresh ones. Simply cook them according to the packages directions and add them to the salad!

Per serving: 253 Calories; 5g Fat (17% calories from fat); 7g Protein; 44g Carbohydrate; 2mg Cholesterol; 319mg Sodium

Savory Broccoli Potato Salad

Serving Size: 8

2 lbs. red potatoes, quartered
1 1/2 c. fresh broccoli florets
1/4 c. fresh orange juice
2 tbsps. extra virgin olive oil
2 tbsps. Dijon mustard
2 tbsps. white wine vinegar
2 tsps. dried whole basil
2 large cloves garlic, minced
2 tbsps. fresh parsley, chopped
2 each green onions, sliced diagonally
  salt to taste

Cook potatoes in boiling water just until tender, about 10-15 minutes. Drain and keep warm. While potatoes are cooking, cook broccoli in boiling water one minute, then drain. Combine broccoli and potatoes and set aside. In a small saucepan, combine juice, Dijon mustard, oil, vinegar, basil and garlic and bring to a boil. Once boiling, remove from heat and pour over potatoes and broccoli. Toss with parsley and onions and serve warm.

Per serving: 126 Calories; 4g Fat (26% calories from fat); 4g Protein; 21g Carbohydrate; 0mg Cholesterol; 60mg Sodium

Spinach and Chicken Salad

Serving Size: 4

Dressing

1/3 c. apple cider vinegar

3 tbsps. water

1 tbsp. olive oil

2 tbsps. Brown sugar replacement

2 tbsps. green onion ,sliced

2 tsps. Dijon mustard

1/2 tsp. salt

1/4 tsp. pepper

Salad

3 bunches fresh spinach, torn and well rinsed

1 1/2 c. cooked chicken breast halves, cubed and chilled

1/2 lb. fresh mushrooms, slices

1 each avocado, peeled and sliced

1/4 c. green onion, sliced

8 oz. water chestnuts, canned and drained

Combine first 8 ingredients for dressing and mix well. Chill at least 30 minutes before serving. Toss together spinach, chicken, mushrooms, avocado, green onion and water chestnuts. Toss with desired amount of dressing immediately before serving.

Per serving: 288 Calories; 15g Fat (46% calories from fat); 25g Protein; 15g Carbohydrate; 60mg Cholesterol; 385mg Sodium

Spinach Salad

Serving Size: 4

1 bunch fresh spinach
1 red onion, sliced
1 large can mandarin oranges, drained
8 oz. fresh mushrooms, sliced

Wash and dry spinach. Toss spinach, onion, mandarin oranges and mushrooms together. Before serving, toss with favorite low calorie dressing.

Per serving: 36 Calories; less than one gram Fat (7% calories from fat); 2g Protein; 8g Carbohydrate; 0mg Cholesterol; 11mg Sodium

Spinach Salad with Curried Dressing

Serving Size: 6

8 c. spinach leaves, washed and torn
1 small red onion, sliced very thin
1 medium Red Delicious apple, chopped
2 tbsps. golden seedless raisins, soaked in hot water
1 tsp. olive oil
1 clove garlic, minced
2 c. lowfat sour cream
1 tbsp. curry powder
1 tbsp. apple juice frozen concentrate
1/2 tsp. ground cardamom
1/4 tsp. cayenne pepper
1/4 tsp. ground ginger

Place spinach in a large bowl, and top with apple, onion rings, and raisins. Place all other ingredients in a blender and blend until smooth. Pour over spinach salad and serve immediately.

Per serving: 156 Calories; 5g Fat (29% calories from fat); 6g Protein; 22g Carbohydrate; 16mg Cholesterol; 136mg Sodium

Tabbouleh

Serving Size: 6

1 c. bulgur
2 medium tomatoes, seeded and chopped
1 medium cucumber, peeled and chopped
5 each green onions, minced
3/4 c. fresh parsley, chopped
1 tbsp. fresh mint, chopped
1 tbsp. olive oil
1/4 tsp. dried whole oregano
1/4 tsp. dried whole basil
1 each lemon juice
 salt and pepper

Wash bulgur wheat in cold water and drain. Add all ingredients to wheat and combine well. Refrigerate until wheat softens. Serve cold.

Notes: Tabbouleh is a Middle-Eastern dish that spotlights bulgur, a wheat that is partially cooked. This salad is great in the summer, and for a fancier presentation, serve it in hollowed out tomatoes.

Per serving: 176 Calories; 3g Fat (14% calories from fat); 7g Protein; 36g Carbohydrate; 0mg Cholesterol; 20mg Sodium

Blue Cheese Dressing

Serving Size: 12

1/2 c. crumbled blue cheese
1 c. plain nonfat yogurt
1 clove minced garlic
1/4 tsp. cracked black pepper
1 tbsp. maltitol

Combine all ingredients and mix well. Cover and refrigerate and let stand one hour before using to allow flavors to blend.

Per serving: 34 Calories; 2g Fat (43% calories from fat); 2g Protein; 3g Carbohydrate; 5mg Cholesterol; 93mg Sodium

Buttermilk Herb Dressing

Serving Size: 16

1 c. low-fat sour cream
3/4 c. low-fat buttermilk
1/4 c. low-fat mayonnaise
2 tbsps. green onions, chopped with tops
1 tbsp. chopped fresh parsley
1/2 tsp. dried dill
1/4 tsp. Worcestershire sauce
1/4 tsp. salt
2 cloves garlic, minced
1 dash hot sauce
3 dashes black pepper

Combine all ingredients, cover and refrigerate at least one hour before serving. Makes 2 cups.

Notes: Buttermilk is a great substitute for whole milk because not only is it rich in flavor, but also lower in fat content.

Per serving: 34 Calories; 2g Fat (50% calories from fat); 1g Protein; 3g Carbohydrate; 5mg Cholesterol; 81mg Sodium

Fat Free Creamy Cucumber Dressing

Serving Size: 12

1 medium cucumber
12 oz. nonfat sour cream
1 tbsp. fresh dill, chopped
1 tbsp. green onions, minced
1/4 tsp. fresh ground black pepper

Peel cucumber and cut in half lengthwise. Scoop out seeds with a teaspoon. Slice cucumbers and place them in a colander. Sprinkle the cucumber with salt and let them sit for a half hour to drain. Rinse cucumbers and squeeze out any excess moisture. Place cucumbers and sour cream in a blender or food processor and blend until smooth. Add herbs and cover and refrigerate. Allow dressing to stand one hour before serving to allow flavors to blend.

Per serving: 24 Calories; less than one gram Fat (2% calories from fat); 2g Protein; 4g Carbohydrate; 4mg Cholesterol; 20mg Sodium

Herbed Vinigrette

Serving Size: 8

1/4 c. white wine vinegar
1/4 tsp. cracked black pepper
1/2 tsp. salt
1 tsp. minced garlic
1 tsp. minced shallots
2 tsps. fresh lemon juice
1 tbsp. Dijon mustard
1/2 c. water
2 tbsps. extra virgin olive oil
1 tsp. minced fresh chives
1 tsp. minced fresh parsley
1 tsp. minced fresh basil

Combine all ingredients, except oil, and shake vigorously. Add oil and shake for one minute. Cover, refrigerate and let stand one hour before using.

Per serving: 34 Calories; 3g Fat (88% calories from fat); 0g Protein; 1g Carbohydrate; 0mg Cholesterol; 158mg Sodium

Oriental Dressing

Serving Size: 16

1/3 c. sesame oil
2 tbsps. rice vinegar
4 tbsps. fresh orange juice
2 tbsps. low sodium soy sauce
2 tbsps. maltitol
1 tsp. minced garlic
1 tbsp. grated ginger root

Combine all ingredients and shake vigorously. Allow to stand, refrigerated, for and hour before using for flavors to blend.

Per serving: 48 Calories; 5g Fat (81% calories from fat); 0g Protein; 2g Carbohydrate; 0mg Cholesterol; 75mg Sodium

Rice and Pasta Dishes

Baked Pasta Primavera

Serving Size: 6

8 oz. pasta, uncooked
1 tsp. olive oil
2 tsps. minced garlic
1 large red bell pepper, roasted and diced
1/2 c. snow peas, trimmed
1/2 c. asparagus, cut in 1" pieces

1/4 c. white wine
1/3 c. green onion, chopped
1 tsp. dried basil
1/4 tsp. ground cumin
1/2 tsp. dried oregano
1 c. cherry tomatoes, halved

Sauce:

2 tsps. butter
1 c. 2% low-fat milk
1/4 tsp. pepper

2 tsps. flour
1/3 c. grated Parmesan cheese

Preheat oven to 400°F. Cook pasta according to package directions, then drain and rinse in cold water. Set aside. In a 10 inch skillet, heat white wine and oil over medium heat and saute asparagus, green onion, garlic, and bell pepper for about 3 minutes. Add spices, cherry tomatoes and snow peas and saute, stirring often, for 2 more minutes. Remove from heat and add to pasta. To make sauce, heat butter over low-medium heat and stir in flour to make a paste. Cook paste for 5 minutes then slowly whisk in milk. Once this mixture is heated, add cheese and pepper. Add sauce to pasta mixture then pour all ingredients into a greased baking dish. Bake about 30 minutes, or until bubbly and golden brown on top.

Per serving: 234 Calories; 5g Fat (21% calories from fat); 10g Protein; 35g Carbohydrate; 11mg Cholesterol; 175mg Sodium

Brown Rice with Vegetables

Serving Size: 6

1/2 c. yellow onions, minced
1/2 c. celery, finely chopped
2 garlic cloves, minced
2 tbsps. canola oil
2 3/4 c. nonfat chicken broth
1 c. long-grain brown rice, rinsed
1 bay leaf
1/4 tsp. salt
1/4 tsp. black pepper, fresh-ground
1/2 c. carrots peeled, diced
1/4 c. green peppers, diced

Saute onion, celery, and garlic in the margarine. In a heavy pan with a tight fitting lid. Add the broth, brown rice, bay leaf, salt and pepper. Cover tightly and cook over low heat for 35-40 minutes. Stir in carrots and green peppers; cook 10-15 minutes longer. Remove bay leaf and fluff with a fork before serving.

Per serving: 178 Calories; 6g Fat (30% calories from fat); 5g Protein; 27g Carbohydrate; 0mg Cholesterol; 265mg Sodium

Creamy Linguini

Serving Size: 6

4 oz. spinach spaghetti or linguini
3 tbsps. skim milk
1 egg, beaten
1/4 c. grated Parmesan cheese
1 tbsp. pimiento, sliced

Cook pasta according to package without the salt or fat. Drain well. Place in large bowl and keep warm. Combine milk and egg in small saucepan. Cook over low heat 1 to 2 minutes, stirring frequently with wire whisk. Add cheese and pimento. Remove from heat. Pour over pasta and toss gently to coat evenly. Serve immediately.

Per serving: 104 Calories; 3g Fat (22% calories from fat); 5g Protein; 15g Carbohydrate; 43mg Cholesterol; 97mg Sodium

Easy Lasagna

Serving Size: 10

10 oz. frozen spinach
60 oz. spaghetti sauce
2 c. nonfat ricotta cheese
1 1/2 c. nonfat mozzarella cheese, shredded
1 egg, beaten
8 oz. lasagna noodles
1/8 tsp. black pepper
1/2 tsp. oregano, optional
1/2 tsp. basil, optional
1 c. water

Thaw the spinach and squeeze dry. In a large container mix the two cheeses, beaten egg, black pepper, oregano and basil. Add the thawed spinach and blend well. Use a 13 x 9 inch pan. Combine water and spaghetti sauce. Put a small amount of the sauce in bottom and spread lightly to cover bottom. Place one third of the uncooked noodles, one third of the sauce and one third of the cheese-spinach mixture. Make 3 layers this way, ending with the sauce. Sprinkle with grated Parmesan cheese if desired. Cover tightly with foil. Bake at 350°F for 1 hour to 1 1/4 hours. Remove foil and continue baking for a few minutes more, until lightly browned and bubbling. Let stand for at least 15 minutes before serving.

Per serving: 343 Calories; 9g Fat (23% calories from fat); 20g Protein; 49g Carbohydrate; 27mg Cholesterol; 1032mg Sodium

Fettuccine Alfredo

Serving Size: 6

12 oz. fettucine, uncooked
3 tbsps. reduced-calorie margarine
1 tbsp. flour
1/2 c. skim milk
1/4 c. Parmesan cheese

Cook fettucine according to package without the salt or fat. Drain well. Place in large bowl and keep warm. Melt margarine in medium saucepan over low heat, add flour. Stir until smooth. Cook 3 to 4 minutes, stirring constantly. Gradually add milk and heat over medium heat. Continue to stir constantly, cook until thickened and bubbly. Reduce to low and add Parmesan cheese. Continue to stir constantly. Cook until cheese melts and sauce is smooth. Pour over fettucine. Toss gently to coat. Serve immediately.

Per serving: 262 Calories; 5g Fat (17% calories from fat); 9g Protein; 44g Carbohydrate; 3mg Cholesterol; 146mg Sodium

Green Rice

Serving Size: 4

1/2 c. green onions, minced
2 tbsps. garlic, minced
1 tsp. extra virgin olive oil
1/4 c. white wine
1/3 c. chopped fresh parsley
1/2 c. spinach leaves, minced
3 c. cooked rice
2 tbsps. pine nuts
2 tbsps. red bell pepper, minced
1/3 c. grated Parmesan cheese

In a 10 inch skillet over medium high heat, heat the olive oil and wine together and saute the garlic and green onion in it for 5 minutes. Add parsley and spinach and cook for 3 more minutes. Add the rice and pine nuts and heat for about 5 minutes, stirring constantly. Remove from heat and stir in bell pepper and cheese.

Per serving: 279 Calories; 6g Fat (20% calories from fat); 9g Protein; 44g Carbohydrate; 7mg Cholesterol; 169mg Sodium

Lean(er) Pesto Sauce with Pasta

Serving Size: 8

3 c. fresh basil, washed and dried
4 garlic cloves, minced
2 tbsps. grated Parmesan cheese
1 c. pine nuts
1/3 c. olive oil
2/3 c. nonfat chicken broth, warmed
8 c. cooked pasta

Chop basil leaves in food processor or blender until finely chopped. Mix the basil with chopped pine nuts, minced garlic and cheese in the processor or blender. While machine is running, slowly pour in a thin stream of oil. Add chicken stock slowly. Continue blending until desired consistency. Toss with pasta. Notes: Pesto sauce should never be heated.

Per serving: 370 Calories; 18g Fat (43% calories from fat); 12g Protein; 43g Carbohydrate; 1mg Cholesterol; 62mg Sodium

Pasta Shells Stuffed With Cheeses

Serving Size: 8

15 oz. nonfat ricotta cheese
1 c. Monterey jack cheese, shredded
2 c. nonfat mozzarella cheese, shredded
1/2 c. grated Parmesan cheese
1/2 c. liquid egg substitute, beaten
10 oz. frozen spinach
1 dash salt
1 dash black pepper
1/2 lb. pasta shells, jumbo size
30 oz. Marinara sauce

Preheat oven to 350°F. Thaw the spinach, chop, and drain very well. Combine the ricotta, jack, Parmesan cheese and 1 cup of the mozzarella cheese. Add the beaten eggs, spinach, salt and pepper. Set aside. Cook pasta according to the package and drain well. Fill the drained and cooled pasta shells with the cheese mixture. Place enough sauce in a pan to just cover bottom. Use a pan large enough to hold the filled shells in one layer. Pour remaining sauce evenly over shells; sprinkle the remaining 1/2 cup mozzarella cheese over top of shells. Bake in preheated 350°F oven for about 30 minutes.

Per serving: 359 Calories; 11g Fat (26% calories from fat); 31g Protein; 39g Carbohydrate; 28mg Cholesterol; 1201mg Sodium

Pasta with Fresh Tomatoes

Serving Size: 4

3/4 pound pasta
3 tbsps. olive oil
2 tbsps. shallots, chopped
3 large tomato, diced
1 tbsp. fresh basil, minced
salt and pepper to taste

Dice the fresh tomatoes. Bring a large pot of water to a rapid boil; add salt if preferred. Drop in the pasta, keeping water boiling rapidly. Cook until tender. DO NOT overcook. Drain well and set aside. Using same large pot, place the olive oil and shallots over medium heat. Cook only until wilted; add tomatoes and cook about 40 seconds. Salt and pepper the mixture to taste. Add the drained pasta and basil and blend well. Serve immediately.

Per serving: 409 Calories; 11g Fat (26% calories from fat); 11g Protein; 64g Carbohydrate; 0mg Cholesterol; 7mg Sodium

Pasta with Pine Nut Garlic Sauce

Serving Size: 6

2 garlic cloves
1/3 c. olive oil
1/3 c. pine nuts
1/4 c. boiling water
1/2 tsp. salt
1/4 tsp. cayenne pepper
6 c. cooked pasta
1 tsp. chopped fresh parsley
2 tbsps. chopped fresh basil
1/2 c. red bell pepper, roasted and diced

Preheat oven to 300°F. Cut the tops off the garlic and brush them with one tsp. olive oil. Place on a baking sheet and roast for 20 minutes or until they are soft. Let them cool, then squeeze the garlic out without the peel. Place the roasted garlic, pine nuts, remaining oil, water, salt, and cayenne pepper in a blender and blend until smooth. Toss the sauce with the hot pasta, herbs and bell pepper and serve.

Notes: To roast a bell pepper, set oven to broil. Place peppers under the broiler and broil until all sides of the pepper are charred, turning as necessary. Remove the peppers when they are black all over then wrap them in plastic. When they have cooled, scrape off the charred skin as much as possible and use.

Per serving: 343 Calories; 16g Fat (43% calories from fat); 8g Protein; 42g Carbohydrate; 0mg Cholesterol; 180mg Sodium

Rice Pilaf

Serving Size: 6

2 tbsps. minced onion
1 tsp. minced garlic
1 tbsp. butter
1 c. long-grain rice
2 c. chicken stock, hot
1 bay leaf
1/2 tsp. dried marjoram
 salt and pepper to taste

Melt the butter over medium heat and add the onion. Cook the onion about 3 minutes, or until it softens. Add the garlic, and cook on minute more. Add rice and stir until all grains are coated with butter, then cook an additional 3 minutes, stirring often. Add remaining ingredients and bring rice to a boil. Once boiling, reduce heat to low and cover. Cook rice covered 15-20 minutes or until water is absorbed and rice is tender. Before serving, stir rice a little to fluff it up and stir back in herbs (remove bay leaf).

Per serving: 135 Calories; 2g Fat (15% calories from fat); 3g Protein; 26g Carbohydrate; 5mg Cholesterol; 751mg Sodium

Risotto

Serving Size: 6

2 tbsps. minced onion
1 tbsp. butter
1 c. Arborio rice
2 1/2 c. chicken stock, hot
1/2 c. white wine, warmed
1/3 c. Parmesan cheese, grated
 salt and pepper to taste

Heat butter in a 2 quart sauce pot until melted over medium heat. Add onions and rice; stir for about 6-8 minutes, or until the rice smells slightly toasted. Add the chicken stock a 1/2 cup at a time, after each addition, stir the rice until the liquid absorbs before adding any more liquid. Add the wine as the last liquid, and stir until the rice is creamy and tender. Add Parmesan and salt and pepper, to taste. Serve warm.

Notes: After you get the basic method of risotto down, try experimenting by adding different herbs, mushrooms, or vegetables.

Per serving: 171 Calories; 3g Fat (20% calories from fat); 4g Protein; 25g Carbohydrate; 9mg Cholesterol; 1016mg Sodium

Saffron Rice and Black Beans

Serving Size: 8

2 c. black beans
1 onion, halved
6 garlic cloves, whole
1/3 tsp. saffron, ground

4 c. nonfat chicken broth
3 bay leaves
2 c. rice

Topping:

6 medium tomatoes, seeded and chopped
2 c. green onions, chopped
2 tbsps. wine vinegar
1/4 tsp. cayenne pepper
black pepper

4 tbsps. olive oil
1 tsp. ground cumin
4 tbsps. fresh parsley

Rinse and sort the beans. Put into a large, heavy pot with lid. Cover with the 4 cups broth. Bring to a boil, cover, and remove from heat. Let stand for 2 hours. Add the halved onions, bay leaves and garlic to beans. Place over low heat and cook, covered, until beans are tender; about 1-1/2 to 2 hours. Check broth and add more if needed while cooking. Remove and discard the onion, bay leaves and garlic cloves. Keep beans warm. Prepare the garnish about 1 hour before serving. Place the tomatoes and onion into a serving bowl. Add the olive oil, vinegar, cumin, cayenne, parsley and black pepper to taste. Toss to blend. Bring 4 cups water to boiling in a heavy saucepan with tight fitting lid. Add the rice and saffron. Stir well, cover, reduce heat and simmer for 20 minutes or until the rice has absorbed all the water. To serve, place the rice, black beans, and the garnish into separate bowls. Guests can serve themselves by placing a serving of rice, topping with the beans and finally with the garnish on their plates.

Per serving: 456 Calories; 9g Fat (17% calories from fat); 18g Protein; 79g Carbohydrate; 0mg Cholesterol; 195mg Sodium

Sandwiches

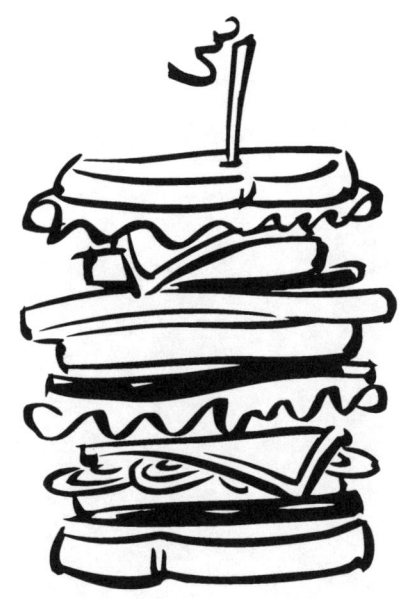

Chicken and Avocado Sandwich

Serving Size: 4

4 boned and skinned chicken breast halves, grilled
4 tbsps. Dijon mustard
4 hamburger buns, mixed grain
2 avocados
1 c. alfalfa sprouts
1 large tomato, sliced

Cut chicken into thin strips, if desired. Spread each bun with Dijon mustard, and top with chicken. Peel, seed, then cut avocado into slices and place 1/2 an avocado on each bun. Top the buns with alfalfa sprouts and tomato slices and serve immediately.

Per serving: 343 Calories; 16g Fat (40% calories from fat); 27g Protein; 26g Carbohydrate; 51mg Cholesterol; 450mg Sodium

Egg Salad Sandwiches

Serving Size: 4

1 1/2 c. egg substitute
1/3 c. fat-free mayonnaise
1 1/2 tsps. Dijon mustard
1/2 c. frozen peas, thawed
1/3 c. bell pepper, chopped
1/3 c. celery, chopped
1/4 c. red onion, finely chopped
1/4 tsp. pepper
 fat-free bread or pita

Cook egg substitute, without stirring, over low heat in skillet that has been prepared with nonstick cooking spray for 18 minutes or until dry. Mix mayonnaise and mustard in medium size bowl. Add peas, bell pepper, celery, onion and pepper. Set aside. Remove eggs from skillet and shop coarsely. Add to vegetables and stir until blended. Spoon onto bread or into pitas.

Per serving: 185 Calories; 10g Fat (50% calories from fat); 12g Protein; 12g Carbohydrate; 2mg Cholesterol; 485mg Sodium

Focaccia Sandwiches

Serving Size: 4

4 pieces focaccia, 4 X 4 squares
4 tbsps. Dijon mustard
1 oz. prosciutto, shaved
1/2 lb. turkey breast slices, sliced thin
2 oz. provolone cheese (4 slices)

Cut each piece of focaccia bread in half to make a top and bottom slice for the sandwiches. Spread the Dijon evenly among the slices and top that with the prosciutto, turkey, and cheese. Place the sandwiches in a 350°F oven and cook until the cheese is melted. Serve immediately.

Notes: If you cannot find prosciutto at the store, you can substitute a very lean cured ham for it.

Per serving: 413 Calories; 12g Fat (27% calories from fat); 27g Protein; 47g Carbohydrate; 38mg Cholesterol; 1585mg Sodium

Grilled Hoagie Sandwiches

Serving Size: 4

1/3 c. fat-free cheddar cheese, shredded
3 tbsps. fat-free mayonnaise
1 tbsp. honey mustard
8 oz. fat-free turkey breast slices
1 large tomato, thinly sliced
1 small onion, thinly sliced
1/2 medium green bell pepper, thinly sliced

In small bowl combine cheese, mayonnaise and mustard. Mix well. Spread 1 tablespoon mustard sauce on each cut side of bread or rolls. Layer with 1/4 each of the turkey, tomato, onion and bell pepper on bottom half. Top with other slice of bread or other side of roll. Wrap in foil. Bake at 450°F for 10 to 15 minutes or until thoroughly heated and cheese is melted.
Serve on French bread rolls, pitas, or fat-free bread.

Per serving: 93 Calories; less than one gram Fat (4% calories from fat); 15g Protein; 8g Carbohydrate; 27mg Cholesterol; 890mg Sodium

Mushroom Cheese Sandwich

Serving Size: 8

1/3 c. fat-free chicken broth
3 tbsps. white wine
2 c. sliced fresh mushrooms
1 red bell pepper, sliced
1 c. green onions, sliced, white only
2 c. fat-free mozzarella cheese, grated
8 slices sourdough bread
spicy mustard to taste

Heat chicken broth and wine in nonstick skillet. Add vegetables and cook until liquid is evaporated. Toast the bread lightly. Spread each bread slice with mustard and top with mushroom mixture. Sprinkle with mozzarella cheese and broil until cheese is melted and bubbly. Serve open face style.

Per serving: 138 Calories; 1g Fat (6% calories from fat); 13g Protein; 19g Carbohydrate; 5mg Cholesterol; 410mg Sodium

Portobello Mushroom Sandwiches

Serving Size: 4

4 large Portobello mushrooms
1 tbsp. olive oil
1/2 tsp. basil
1/2 tsp. oregano
1/4 tsp. garlic powder
salt and pepper to taste
4 hamburger buns, mixed grain
4 tbsps. pesto sauce

To clean mushrooms, remove the stem and wash the excess dirt off the cap. Turn the cap upside down and use a teaspoon to scrape off as much of the black ribs as you can. Combine olive oil and spices and brush caps with mixture. Heat a nonstick skillet over medium high heat and cook the whole caps about 5 minutes on each side, or until tender. While mushrooms are cooking, toast buns in a moderate oven. After buns are toasted, spread one tablespoon of pesto sauce on each bun. When mushroom is done, place on the bun and serve hot.

Notes: This sandwich can be served like a regular hamburger, with lettuce and tomatoes, if you wish.

Per serving: 229 Calories; 13g Fat (50% calories from fat); 7g Protein; 22g Carbohydrate; 4mg Cholesterol; 301mg Sodium

Roasted Corn y Salsa Pita Sandwiches

Serving Size: 6

Sandwiches:

4 ears corn

1 red bell pepper, chopped

6 bacon slices, cooked

1 1/2 c. nonfat cheddar cheese, shredded

1 1/2 c. shredded red cabbage

1 tomato, chopped

6 pitas

Salsa:

1 c. low-fat sour cream

2 tbsps. chopped onions

1 tsp. chili powder

1/4 tsp. salt

3 tbsps. lime juice

1 garlic clove, minced

1 tsp. ground cumin

1/4 tsp. cayenne pepper

SALSA: Mix all the salsa ingredients well and chill.

SANDWICHES:

Place corn, husk and all, in an oven that has been preheated to 400°F. Roast in the oven for 15-20 minutes, or until the corn is tender. Let corn cool until you can hold it, and cut corn from cob. Combine corn, finely shredded cabbage, green pepper, tomato and cooked crumbled bacon in a large bowl. Stir in 3/4 cup of the salsa mix, blending well. Cover and chill mixture. When ready to serve, fill pita bread with corn mixture, top with remaining salsa and shredded cheese.

Per serving: 351 Calories; 7g Fat (17% calories from fat); 21g Protein; 53g Carbohydrate; 18mg Cholesterol; 775mg Sodium

Seafood Salad Sandwich

Serving Size: 2

2 c. crab surimi seafood chunks, flake-style
1/2 c. fat-free mayonnaise
2 stalks celery, chopped
3 tbsps. onion, finely chopped
fat-free bread or pita

Cut crab flakes in half or shred. Combine with remaining ingredients, except bread. Serve on bread or in pita.

Per serving: 294 Calories; 2g Fat (7% calories from fat); 36g Protein; 31g Carbohydrate; 71mg Cholesterol; 1130mg Sodium

Veggie Pita Sandwiches

Serving Size: 4

4 pita bread rounds
1 c. broccoli florets, chopped
1 c. carrots, thinly sliced
1 c. mushrooms, thinly sliced
3 green onions, thinly sliced
4 tbsps. fat-free ranch salad dressing
1 c. alfalfa sprouts

Combine broccoli, carrots, mushrooms and green onions in microwave-proof dish. Cover with plastic wrap; vent. Cook 6 to 8 minutes on high or until vegetables are tender. Cover pitas with paper towels and heat on high for 1 minute or until heated thoroughly. Cut each pita in half and stuff with vegetable mixture; top with alfalfa sprouts and ranch dressing. Serve immediately.

Per serving: 244 Calories; 1g Fat (4% calories from fat); 10g Protein; 50g Carbohydrate; 0mg Cholesterol; 492mg Sodium

Meat Dishes

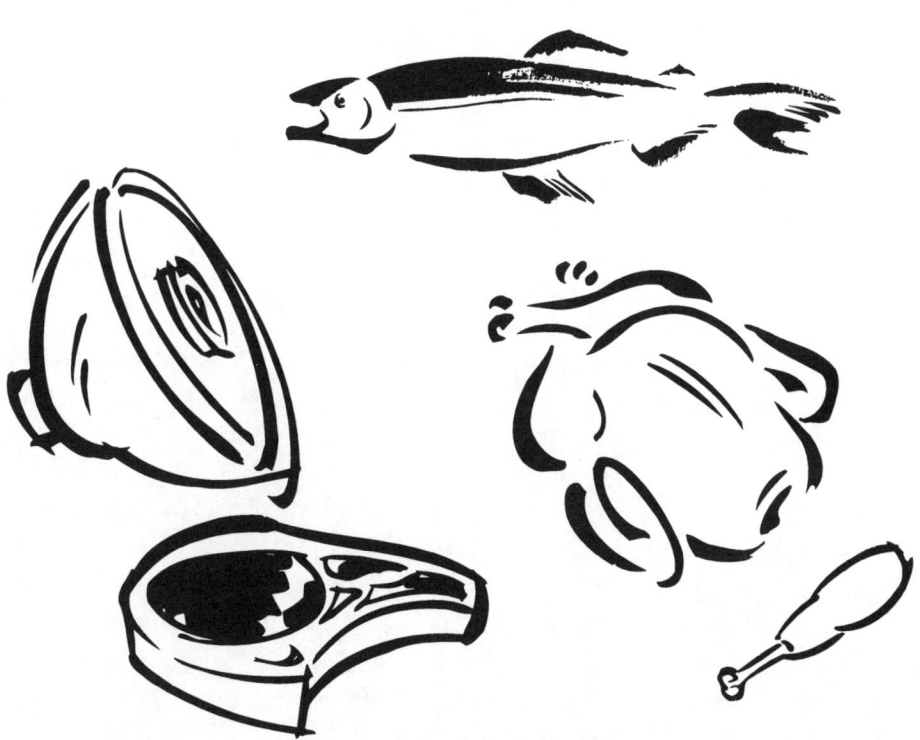

Beef and Cornbread Casserole

Serving Size: 8

1 lb. extra lean ground beef
1 tsp. dried oregano
3/4 c. salsa
8 oz. tomato sauce
16 oz. canned corn, drained
1/2 c. nonfat cheddar cheese
8 oz. corn muffins mix

Preheat oven to 375°F. In 10 inch skillet over medium high heat, cook beef and oregano until beef is browned, stirring frequently to break up meat. Pour off any fat. Add salsa, tomato sauce and corn. Reduce heat to low and bring to a simmer. Stir in cheese and pour in a 2 quart casserole dish. Prepare corn muffin mix according to package directions, spread over meat mixture. Bake 25-30 minutes or until cornbread is deep golden brown and pulls away from the edges of the dish. Allow to stand 10 minutes before serving.

Per serving: 291 Calories; 13g Fat (39% calories from fat); 17g Protein; 28g Carbohydrate; 55mg Cholesterol; 580mg Sodium

Beef in Mushroom Sauce

Serving Size: 4

3/4 lb. lean beef (boneless round steak)
2 1/2 c. fresh mushrooms, sliced
1/2 c. onion, chopped
3 cloves garlic, minced
1/4 c. dry red wine
2 tbsps. cornstarch
10 1/2 oz. beef broth, condensed
1/4 tsp. pepper
3/4 c. low-fat sour cream
2 c. cooked rice hot
2 tbsps. fresh parsley, chopped

Trim fat from beef steak. Cut beef with the grain into 2 inch strips then cut the strips diagonally across the grain into 1/4 inch slices. Spray a 10 inch nonstick pan with vegetable oil cooking spray then heat over medium high heat. Stir beef, mushrooms, onion and garlic into the skillet. Cook for about five minutes, or until beef is cooked, then stir in wine. Heat to boiling, then cover and reduce heat to a simmer. Simmer 10 minutes. Stir cornstarch into beef broth until the cornstarch is completely dissolved. Stir into beef, and cook until thickened and boiling. Allow to boil for one minute. Stir in sour cream and pepper and bring to a simmer. Cover and gently simmer for 30 minutes, or until beef is tender, stirring occasionally. Stir in parsley and serve over hot rice.

Per serving: 418 Calories; 16g Fat (35% calories from fat); 23g Protein; 41g Carbohydrate; 62mg Cholesterol; 574mg Sodium

Hearty Beef Casserole

Serving Size: 8

1 lb. extra lean ground beef, browned and drained
1 c. chopped onions
28 oz. canned tomatoes, chopped
1 tbsp. Worcestershire sauce
1 tsp. salt
2 c. potatoes, diced
1/3 c. all-purpose flour
10 oz. frozen corn, thawed
2 c. canned pinto beans, rinsed and drained
1 large bell pepper, cut in strips
1 1/2 c. nonfat cheddar cheese, shredded

Preheat oven to 375°F. In a bowl, combine browned and drained beef, onion, and tomatoes with liquid, Worcestershire sauce and salt. Spoon into a greased 3 quart casserole. Layer the potatoes, flour, corn, pinto beans and green peppers on top. Cover and bake for 45 minutes. Sprinkle with the cheese and continue baking, uncovered, for 30 minutes longer.

Per serving: 327 Calories; 11g Fat (28% calories from fat); 24g Protein; 36g Carbohydrate; 43mg Cholesterol; 940mg Sodium

Herbed Pot Roast

Serving Size: 10

3 lbs. beef pot roast (boneless rump roast)
1/2 tsp. cracked black pepper
2 cloves garlic, minced
1 c. dry red wine
1 1/2 c. beef broth
1/4 c. fresh parsley, chopped
1 tsp. dried thyme
5 whole cloves
3 each bay leaves
10 new potatoes
5 medium carrots
2 medium onions, cut into eighths

Trim all fat from the outside of the roast. Combine pepper and garlic and rub it all over the roast. Place roast in a very large pot that has a lid. Add wine, broth, parsley, thyme, cloves, and bay leaves. Heat to boiling, then reduce heat to a simmer. Lower and simmer 2 1/2 hours. Turn roast over in the pot. Add remaining ingredients and any additional beef broth if necessary. Cover and simmer about one more hour or until beef and vegetables are tender. Remove cloves and bay leaves before serving, and serve the roast and vegetables with the juices it was cooked in.

Notes: When cooking tougher pieces of meats for a long time to ensure a tender piece, a great way to test if the meat is done is to insert a knife into the roast, and if it is done, it will come out without any resistance.

Per serving: 412 Calories; 23g Fat (51% calories from fat); 24g Protein; 24g Carbohydrate; 79mg Cholesterol; 344mg Sodium

Microwave Meatloaf

Serving Size: 6

1 1/2 pounds extra lean ground beef
3/4 c. chopped onions
2 cloves minced garlic
1/2 c. bread crumbs
1 large egg
2 tbsps. ketchup
2/3 c. skim milk
1/8 tsp. paprika
 salt and pepper to taste

Mix together the beef, onion, garlic, bread crumbs, beaten egg, ketchup, milk and seasonings. Press mixture into a 9-inch glass pie plate or similar microwave-safe dish. Spread about 2 tablespoons ketchup evenly over top of meat. If your microwave has a temperature probe, insert it so tip is in center of food. Cover tightly with plastic wrap, arranging loosely around probe to vent. Microwave on medium high for 26-28 minutes, or until probe reaches 170°F. Let meat loaf stand for 10 minutes before serving. If not using a probe, insert meat thermometer to check doneness.

Per serving: 336 Calories; 21g Fat (57% calories from fat); 24g Protein; 11g Carbohydrate; 109mg Cholesterol; 235mg Sodium

Peppered Beef Tenderloin

Serving Size: 4

3/4 lb. beef tenderloin
1/2 tsp. dried marjoram
2 tsps. coarsely ground pepper
1 tbsp. margarine
1 c. fresh mushrooms, sliced
1 small onion, thinly sliced
3/4 c. beef broth
1/4 c. dry red wine
1 tbsp. cornstarch

Trim fat from the tenderloin, then cut it into four equal steaks, each about 3/4 inch thick. Combine marjoram and pepper and rub this on all sides of the steaks. Heat a 10 inch pan over medium heat and add the margarine. When the pan is hot, add the steaks and cook each one 4-5 minutes on each side, turning once. Remove beef from the pan, set aside, but keep them warm. Cook mushrooms and onions in the same skillet about five minutes. Combine beef broth, wine and cornstarch until the cornstarch is dissolved. Pour mixture into the skillet and stir constantly until it thickens and boils. Allow to boil for one minute, pour sauce over beef and serve.
Notes: This dish is great served over rice or egg noodles.

Per serving: 311 Calories; 23g Fat (69% calories from fat); 16g Protein; 7g Carbohydrate; 60mg Cholesterol; 379mg Sodium

Stuffed Cabbage

Serving Size: 8

1 head cabbage
1 egg white
1 onion
1 1/2 lbs. ground beef, extra lean
3/4 cup cooked rice
Seasonings of your choice such as garlic,
 caraway or fennel

Separate cabbage leaves from head and boil them until tender, about 6 minutes. In medium bowl, combine all ingredients except cabbage. Season to taste. Put small amount of stuffing in cabbage leaves. Roll. Put cabbage rolls in heated frying pan coated with nonstick cooking spray. Cover and cook until brown. Turn over and continue to cook until brown.

Per serving: 247 Calories; 15g Fat (54% calories from fat); 18g Protein; 10g Carbohydrate; 59mg Cholesterol; 82mg Sodium

Veal and Apple Scaloppine

Serving Size: 6

1 lb. veal cutlets, pounded thin
2 medium Granny Smith apples
1 tbsp. shallots, minced
1 tbsp. butter
1/2 c. Calvados
1/2 c. light cream

Preheat oven to 350°F. Pound slices of veal between two pieces of plastic with the flat side of a meat mallet until the veal is very thin (it can also be purchased this way). Peel, core and slice the apples.

Spray a medium sized baking dish with nonstick cooking spray and spread the apple slices over the bottom of the dish. Bake uncovered for 20 minutes.

In a large skillet over medium high heat, melt the butter and lightly brown each piece of veal on both sides. Place the veal on top of the baked apple slices as they come out of the pan.

After all the veal has cooked, add shallots to the pan and saute them for 3 minutes. Pour Calvados into the pan and scrape any brown pieces off the bottom of the pan. Add the cream and cook over medium heat for 5 minutes. Pour sauce over veal and apples. Bake veal until bubbling, about 15 minutes.

Per serving: 231 Calories; 11g Fat (52% calories from fat); 16g Protein; 6g Carbohydrate; 82mg Cholesterol; 91mg Sodium

Veal and Fettucine Florentine

Serving Size: 4

3/4 lb. veal cubes from round steak
1 c. fresh mushrooms, sliced
1/4 c. shallots, chopped
1/2 c. white wine
1/2 c. beef broth
2 tsps. cornstarch
1/8 tsp. pepper
10 oz. frozen chopped spinach, thawed and drained
4 c. fettucine, cooked and hot

Spray 10 inch skillet with vegetable oil cooking spray and heat pan over medium high heat. Saute veal, mushrooms, and shallots for about five minutes, or until veal is done. Combine wine, broth, cornstarch and pepper, then stir it into the skillet and add the spinach. Heat until mixture boils, stirring constantly. Lower heat and simmer five minutes, then pour over fettucine and serve.

Per serving: 466 Calories; 4g Fat (8% calories from fat); 31g Protein; 70g Carbohydrate; 72mg Cholesterol; 328mg Sodium

Baked Fish With Vegetables

Serving Size: 4

1 lb. cod fillets
1 tbsp. canola oil
1 c. onions, sliced
3 c. zucchini, sliced
1 c. red bell peppers, sliced
3/4 c. chopped tomatoes, without seeds
3 tbsps. white wine, optional
1 tbsp. lemon juice
1/2 tsp. salt
1/2 tsp. ground basil
1/4 tsp. black pepper, freshly ground
1 dash hot pepper sauce
1/4 c. grated Parmesan cheese

Place fillets in a layer in greased 9-inch baking dish. Saute onion, zucchini and red pepper in oil over medium heat until crisp-tender, about 6-8 minutes; spoon over fillets. Top with tomatoes.

Combine wine, lemon juice, salt, basil, pepper and pepper sauce; pour over fillets.

Bake, uncovered, in preheated 350°F oven for 25-30 minutes. Remove vegetables and fish to heated platter. Sprinkle with Parmesan cheese. Serve over rice. Pour pan juices over fish and vegetables if desired.

Per serving: 206 Calories; 6g Fat (29% calories from fat); 25g Protein; 11g Carbohydrate; 54mg Cholesterol; 454mg Sodium

Baked Halibut

Serving Size: 6

1 1/2 lbs. halibut fillets
1/2 tsp. salt
1/4 tsp. paprika
1/4 tsp. pepper
1 red bell pepper, cut in rings
1 tomato, sliced
1 onion, sliced
2 tbsps. lime juice
2 tbsps. olive oil
1 garlic clove, minced
2 limes, cut into wedges

Cut fish into serving-sized pieces. Place in ovenproof baking dish. Sprinkle with salt, paprika and pepper. Top with red pepper rings, tomato slices and onion slices. Mix lime juice, oil and garlic. Pour over the fish fillets. Cover and bake 15 minutes at 375°F. Uncover and bake about 10-13 minutes longer or until fish flakes easily. Serve with lime wedges.

Per serving: 187 Calories; 7g Fat (35% calories from fat); 24g Protein; 6g Carbohydrate; 36mg Cholesterol; 241mg Sodium

Broiled Sole with Cheese

Serving Size: 6

2 lbs. sole fillets or red snapper

Topping:

1/3 c. low-fat mayonnaise

1/3 c. grated Parmesan cheese

1/4 c. green onion, minced

1/2 tsp. garlic powder

1/2 tsp. dried whole basil

Preheat oven to 350°F. Place fish in a ovenproof glass baking dish sprayed with nonstick cooking spray and bake 8 minutes or until fish flakes easily with a fork. While the fish is cooking, combine ingredients for topping. Spread topping evenly over the cooked fish fillets. Set oven to broil and broil 6 inches from heat for 5 minutes or until topping is golden brown.

Per serving: 166 Calories; 6g Fat (34% calories from fat); 25g Protein; 2g Carbohydrate; 9mg Cholesterol; 252mg Sodium

Broiled Swordfish with Mango Salsa

Serving Size: 4

Mango Salsa:
2 each jalapenos, seeded and chopped
3 tbsps. orange juice
2 tbsps. green onions, chopped (with top)
2 tbsps. chopped fresh cilantro
1/4 tsp. salt
2 c. mangos, peeled and chopped

Swordfish:
4 swordfish steaks
1/4 c. lime juice
1/4 c. orange juice
1 tbsp. grated lime rind
1/2 tsp. salt
1 clove garlic, minced

To make salsa, combine all ingredients, cover and refrigerate. Place steaks in a plastic bag with remaining ingredients and refrigerate for 2 hours.

Set oven to broil. Spray broiler rack with nonstick cooking spray. Remove fish from marinade and place the fish on rack in the broiler pan. Broil with steaks about inches from heat about 15 minutes, turning the steaks after 8 minutes. Fish is done when it flakes easily with fork. Serve with a dollop of salsa on top.

Notes: Mangos are ripe when the flesh is soft and the color is mostly reddish-orange.

Per serving: 269 Calories; 7g Fat (24% calories from fat); 35g Protein; 16g Carbohydrate; 66mg Cholesterol; 556mg Sodium

Fettuccine with Shrimp

Serving Size: 4

8 oz. fettucine, uncooked
1 1/2 c. chicken broth
1/4 c. white wine
1/4 tsp. dried marjoram
salt and pepper to taste
3/4 lb. shrimp, peeled and deveined
1 tbsp. cornstarch
1 c. 1% low-fat milk
1/4 c. Swiss cheese, grated
2 tbsps. green onions, minced

Cook pasta according to package directions, drain and set aside to keep warm. Combine chicken broth, wine, marjoram and salt and pepper in a saucepan and bring to a boil. Add shrimp and return mixture to a boil. Cook one minute or until shrimp are opaque. Remove shrimp from sauce and set aside to keep warm. Bring broth to a full boil and boil until mixture is reduced to 1/2 cup. Combine cornstarch and milk and stir until cornstarch is dissolved. Add cornstarch mixture to boiling broth, stirring constantly. Bring mixture back to a boil, and boil one minute, stirring constantly. Add cheese and onions and stir until cheese is melted. Return shrimp to saucepan and heat until shrimp are completely hot again. Serve over the hot fettuccine.

Per serving: 386 Calories; 6g Fat (15% calories from fat); 29g Protein; 49g Carbohydrate; 139mg Cholesterol; 767mg Sodium

Flounder Baked in Lettuce Leaves

Serving Size: 4

1 head romaine lettuce
1 1/2 lbs. flounder fillets
1/2 cup fresh parsley, finely chopped
1 c. chopped onions
1 carrot, grated
1/2 c. white wine
salt and pepper to taste

Preheat oven to 400°F. Remove and wash 8-10 large leaves from the romaine lettuce. Line the bottom and sides of a baking dish with leaves, allowing the leaves to hang over edge of dish. Place 1 fillet into dish; cover with onion, carrot and parsley. Sprinkle with a little salt and black pepper. Place the second fillet on top of the first. Fold the ends of the lettuce leaves over top fillet. Add wine to the dish. Cover dish tightly with foil and bake for 15 minutes. Remove foil, fold back the lettuce leaves and serve immediately.

Per serving: 181 Calories; 1g Fat (7% calories from fat); 28g Protein; 9g Carbohydrate; 0mg Cholesterol; 118mg Sodium

Ginger Grilled Fish

Serving Size: 4

4 swordfish steaks
1/4 c. lime juice
2 tbsps. canola oil
1 tsp. Dijon mustard
2 tsps. fresh ginger root, grated
1/2 tsp. salt
1/4 tsp. cayenne pepper
black pepper

In a bowl, combine the lime juice, 1 tablespoon oil, ginger, cayenne pepper and enough freshly ground black pepper to suit your taste. Marinate the fish in the marinade for 45-60 minutes. Turn steaks 2-3 times. Have the grill prepared with white coals and brush the cooking grill with the remaining one tablespoon oil. Grill the fish until cooked through and opaque in the center. Turn fish after about 4-5 minutes. Total grilling time will depend on your grill and the heat of the coals.

* To broil instead, use a broiler pan brushed with oil and broil until center is opaque. Will take about 10 minutes total in broiler. Turn steaks after 5 minutes, and baste often with marinade.

Per serving: 272 Calories; 14g Fat (47% calories from fat); 34g Protein; 2g Carbohydrate; 66mg Cholesterol; 436mg Sodium

Gingered Dijon Salmon

Serving Size: 4

4 tbsps. grated ginger root
8 tsps. Dijon mustard
2 tbsps. brown sugar replacement
2 tbsps. fresh lemon juice
1/4 tsp. black pepper
20 oz. salmon steaks

In a small mixing bowl, combine the first five ingredients. Brush both sides of the salmon steaks with the mixture. Cover and refrigerate one hour. Grill fish over medium hot coals, turning once, until fish flakes easily with a fork, or broil 6 inches from heat in oven 6-8 minutes more, or until done.

Per serving: 178 Calories; 5g Fat (28% calories from fat); 29g Protein; 2g Carbohydrate; 74mg Cholesterol; 221mg Sodium

Italian Baked Halibut

Serving Size: 4

4 halibut steaks or fillets
1/4 c. white wine
3 tbsps. ripe olives, chopped
1 tbsp. capers
4 each anchovy fillets, drained and chopped
2 cloves garlic, minced
28 oz. Italian plum tomatoes, drained and chopped
1 tsp. dried basil

Preheat oven to 350°F. Place steaks or fillets in an ungreased baking dish. Mix remaining ingredients and pour them over fish. Bake uncovered for about 35 minutes or until the fish flakes easily with a fork.

Per serving: 255 Calories; 6g Fat (21% calories from fat); 38g Protein; 10g Carbohydrate; 58mg Cholesterol; 335mg Sodium

Italian Fish in Foil Packets

Serving Size: 4

2 tbsps. minced onions	3/4 c. white wine
1 tsp. minced garlic	1/2 c. fresh mushrooms, sliced
1 tbsp. cornstarch	1/3 c. water
2 tbsps. lemon juice	2 tbsps. chopped parsley
1/2 tsp. black pepper	1/4 tsp. salt

1/2 lb. flounder fillets
1 c. shrimp, peeled and deveined
16 oz. Italian plum tomatoes, drained

Spray an 8 inch skillet with nonstick cooking spray and heat over medium heat. Add onions and saute until tender. Add garlic and saute until aromatic, about one minute. Add wine and mushrooms and cook until mushrooms are tender. Combine cornstarch and water and stir until cornstarch is dissolved, then stir it into mushroom mix. Cook, stirring constantly, until mixture comes to a boil. After it has come to a boil, stir for one minute more, then stir in tomatoes lemon juice, parsley, pepper and salt. Place equal potions of fish on 4 pieces of heavy aluminum foil. Divide the shrimp and tomato sauce mixture evenly among the 4 pieces of foil. Seal foil packets and place on grill 4-6 inches from medium hot coals. Cook for 15 minutes or until fish flakes easily with a fork.

Notes: These foil packets can be cooked in the oven also - bake at 400°F for 15-20 minutes or until fish flakes easily with a fork.

Per serving: 133 Calories; 1g Fat (9% calories from fat); 15g Protein; 9g Carbohydrate; 38mg Cholesterol; 216mg Sodium

Poached Sole with Tarragon

Serving Size: 4

1 1/2 lbs. sole fillets
1 tbsp. butter
1/2 c. chopped green onions
1/4 tsp. tarragon, dried
2/3 c. low sodium chicken broth
 salt and pepper to taste
 lemon wedges, optional

Rinse fish and pat dry. In large heavy skillet, melt butter over medium heat. Add chopped onions and tarragon leaves. Cook until onions are soft - about 3 minutes. Add broth and bring to a boil. Place fish in single layer in this mixture. Reduce heat, cover, and simmer until just translucent, about 5-7 minutes. Fish is done when it flakes easily with a fork. Carefully remove fish from pan, place on serving plate and keep warm. Turn heat to high and allow the juices in pan to cook until reduced to about one half. Pour juice over fish and immediately serve with lemon wedges and salt and pepper if desired.

Per serving: 148 Calories; 4g Fat (23% calories from fat); 27g Protein; 1g Carbohydrate; 8mg Cholesterol; 213mg Sodium

Scallops with Roasted Red Pepper Coulis

Serving Size: 4

2 large red bell peppers
1/4 tsp. salt
1 tsp. hot sauce
2 cloves garlic, minced
3 oz. lowfat cream cheese, cut into pieces
1 lb. scallops
1/2 bunch chives, chopped fine

Set oven to broil. When heated, place red bell peppers under heat and broil until skin is charred, turning as necessary. After all sides are evenly charred, take out peppers and wrap them in plastic. After peppers have cooled off, remove the plastic and scrape the black charred skin off the peppers as much as possible. Remove stem and seeds from the pepper and place them in a food processor or blender with the salt, hot sauce, and garlic and blend until very smooth. Place the pepper puree in a sauce pan over medium heat and heat until hot. Stir in cream cheese, stirring constantly just until melted. Remove from heat, then set aside the sauce, but keep it warm. Spray a 10 inch skillet with nonstick cooking spray. Heat over medium high heat then add scallops and stir fry them for about five minutes or until they are white in the center. Serve the scallops in a pool of the red pepper coulis and sprinkle with chives before serving.

Per serving: 163 Calories; 5g Fat (28% calories from fat); 22g Protein; 6g Carbohydrate; 49mg Cholesterol; 468mg Sodium

Shrimp Quesadillas

Serving Size: 4

8 flour tortillas
1 lb. shrimp, cooked
1 1/2 c. lowfat cheddar cheese, grated
2 tbsps. chopped fresh cilantro
1/2 c. chopped tomatoes

Place four tortillas on the counter and top each with a little cheese, then the shrimp, cilantro and tomatoes, and then a little more cheese. Top each with another tortilla and place in a skillet over medium high heat. Turn tortilla when lightly brown on one side and brown the other side. Cut into wedges and serve hot.

Per serving: 470 Calories; 14g Fat (27% calories from fat); 44g Protein; 42g Carbohydrate; 242mg Cholesterol; 851mg Sodium

Stuffed Red Snapper

Serving Size: 6

4 lbs. whole red snapper, cleaned	1 tsp. salt
1 yellow onion, diced	2 celery stalks, diced
2 tbsps. butter	1/2 c. bell peppers, chopped
4 c. soft bread crumbs	1/2 c. low-fat sour cream
1 lemon, chopped	2 tbsps. lemon zest, grated
1 tsp. black pepper	1 tsp. paprika

Preheat oven to 350°F. Grate the yellow part of the lemon for the zest, set aside. Peel the lemon and remove any seeds. Chop the fruit of the lemon, set aside. Wash fish under cold running water, taking care to wash inside thoroughly. Dry completely. Sprinkle inside with 1/2 teaspoon salt and set aside while preparing stuffing. Melt butter in skillet; add onions, celery and green peppers. Saute until onions are soft and translucent. Add remaining 1/2 teaspoon salt and the remaining ingredients. Blend well. Stuff the fish cavity loosely; fasten with metal skewers and use string to tie securely. Spray a baking dish or pan large with nonstick cooking spray that is large enough so fish won't be crowded. Place fish in pan and bake in preheated 350°F oven for 35-40 minutes. Baste with vegetable oil every 7-8 minutes until fish flakes easily. Remove the skewers and allow to set for about 5 minutes. Serve immediately.

Per serving: 455 Calories; 10g Fat (21% calories from fat); 66g Protein; 22g Carbohydrate; 126mg Cholesterol; 776mg Sodium

Lamb with Garlic and Rosemary

Serving Size: 4

4 lamb cutlets
1 tbsp. extra virgin olive oil
1/2 tsp. garlic powder
1/2 tsp. dried rosemary powder
 salt and pepper to taste

Lightly season lamb with salt and pepper. Combine garlic and rosemary and sprinkle over lamb cutlets on both sides. Heat olive oil in a pan large enough to hold all cutlets over medium high heat. Once pan is hot, place lamb in the pan and cook quickly, about 3 minutes on each side for a medium done lamb, a little longer for well-done. Serve immediately.

Per serving: 183 Calories; 9g Fat (48% calories from fat); 23g Protein; 0g Carbohydrate; 74mg Cholesterol; 74mg Sodium

Lamb with Mint Sauce

Serving Size: 4

2/3 c. plain nonfat yogurt
1/4 c. cucumber, peeled and shredded
1/4 c. fresh mint leaves, firmly packed
2 tbsps. maltitol
4 lamb loin chops

Place yogurt, cucumber, mint and maltitol in blender or food processor and blend until smooth.

Set oven to broil. Spray broiler pan with non-stick cooking spray. Trim all excess fat from lamb chops and place them on the broiler pan. Broil with tops of steaks 2-3 inches from heat for 10-12 minutes, turning lamb after 5 minutes. Serve with sauce (sauce should be room temperature).

Per serving: 321 Calories; 24g Fat (68% calories from fat); 17g Protein; 9g Carbohydrate; 68mg Cholesterol; 80mg Sodium

Pecan Crusted Lamb Chops

Serving Size: 6

6 lamb cutlets
1 c. barbecue sauce
1 c. chopped pecans
 salt and pepper to taste

Set oven to broil. Season lamb cutlets with salt and pepper and brush generously with barbecue sauce. Press each cutlet into the chopped pecans on both sides. Broil lamb 6 inches from heat about 3-4 minutes on each side or until the lamb is done to your liking. Serve with additional barbecue sauce, if desired.

Per serving: 247 Calories; 13g Fat (49% calories from fat); 24g Protein; 7g Carbohydrate; 74mg Cholesterol; 413mg Sodium

Black Bean and Pork Stew

Serving Size: 4

4 c. water
2 each ancho chilies
1 1/2 c. chopped tomatoes, peeled and seeded
1/2 c. dry red wine
1 tsp. dried marjoram
1/2 tsp. cumin
1/4 tsp. ground cinnamon
2 tbsps. cilantro, chopped
1 medium red bell pepper, cut into 1 inch pieces
1/2 c. dried black beans
3/4 lb. pork shoulder, boneless
1/2 c. chopped onion
1 tsp. dried sage
1/2 tsp. salt
1/2 tsp. chili powder
3 cloves garlic minced
2 c. butternut squash, peeled and cut into 1 inch cubes

Heat water, beans and chilies to boiling in a large sauce pot. Boil uncovered for five minutes, cover and remove form heat then let stand for one hour. Remove chilies and set aside for later. Heat beans to boiling, then reduce heat and simmer covered for one hour, or until beans are almost done. Seed and coarsely chop chilies. Trim fat from pork and cut into one inch cubes. Stir in pork, chilies, and remaining ingredients except squash, bell pepper, and cilantro into beans. Cover and simmer 30 minutes, stirring occasionally. Stir in squash, and simmer 30 more minutes. Stir in bell pepper and simmer five more minutes, then add cilantro and serve.

Per serving: 346 Calories; 12g Fat (34% calories from fat); 19g Protein; 35g Carbohydrate; 45mg Cholesterol; 355mg Sodium

Ham with Cabbage and Apples

Serving Size: 4

4 c. shredded cabbage
1/2 c. chopped onion
1 tbsp. brown sugar replacement
1 tbsp. cider vinegar
1 pinch cinnamon
1/8 tsp. pepper
1 large Granny Smith apple, peeled and sliced thin
4 each extra lean ham steaks

Spray 10 inch nonstick skillet with vegetable oil spray and saute cabbage and onion until both are soft. Add remaining ingredients and cook until ham is hot, about 15 minutes.

Per serving: 318 Calories; 10g Fat (29% calories from fat); 46g Protein; 10g Carbohydrate; 102mg Cholesterol; 2892mg Sodium

Pork Chops in Apple Juice

Serving Size: 4

4 pork center loin chops
1/4 tsp. dried sage
salt and pepper to taste
1 c. apple juice, no sugar added
1/4 c. golden raisins
1/4 c. chopped pecans
2 tbsps. green onion, minced

Preheat oven to 350°F. Trim any excess fat from pork chops and brown them in a skillet sprayed with nonstick cooking spray. Arrange single layer in an ovenproof baking dish and sprinkle the chops with sage, salt and pepper, and raisins. Add the apple juice, cover and bake about one hour, or until meat is tender. Garnish with pecans and green onion.

Per serving: 309 Calories; 17g Fat (49% calories from fat); 23g Protein; 16g Carbohydrate; 75mg Cholesterol; 71mg Sodium

Pork with Creamy Basil Sauce

Serving Size: 4

3/4 lb. pork tenderloin
1 tsp. vegetable oil
1/4 c. fresh basil, chopped
1/4 c. chicken broth
3 oz. low-fat cream cheese
1/8 tsp. cayenne pepper
4 cloves garlic, minced
pinch white pepper

Trim fat from pork tenderloin. Cut pork across into 8 pieces, then flatten each to a 1/4 inch thick piece by placing each piece between plastic wrap and pounding them with the flat side of a meat mallet. Cook pork quickly in oil in a 10 inch skillet over medium high heat about three minutes on each side. Stir in remaining ingredients and reduce heat to medium and stir constantly until cheese is melted. Cover and simmer about 5 minutes then serve.

Per serving: 168 Calories; 8g Fat (45% calories from fat); 20g Protein; 2g Carbohydrate; 67mg Cholesterol; 289mg Sodium

South Seas Casserole

Serving Size: 6

13 1/2 oz. pineapple chunks in juice	3 c. extra lean ham, cubed
1/3 c. brown sugar replacement	2 c. canned sweet potatoes, cooked and sliced
1/4 c. all-purpose flour	1/4 tsp. curry powder
1/8 tsp. black pepper	2 tbsps. vinegar
3/4 c. water	

Topping:

1 c. all-purpose flour	2 tsps. maltitol
2 tsps. baking powder	1/4 tsp. salt
1/2 c. macadamia nuts, chopped	2 large eggs
1/2 c. skim milk	2 tbsps. margarine, melted
1/2 tsp. ground cinnamon, optional	

Drain pineapple and reserve syrup. Layer pineapple chunks, cubed ham and sliced cooked sweet potatoes in a 2-quart casserole. Combine brown sugar replacement substitute, flour, curry powder and pepper. Blend in the reserved pineapple juice, water and vinegar. Pour mixture over casserole. Bake in preheated 375°F oven for 20 minutes. Cover with topping and bake 20-25 minutes longer or until golden brown.

Topping:
Combine flour, baking powder, salt, cinnamon (if desired) and chopped nuts. Beat egg yolks until creamy. Stir in milk, maltitol and margarine. Add dry ingredients and stir just until dry particles are moistened. Beat egg whites until stiff then fold into batter.

Per serving: 390 Calories; 12g Fat (27% calories from fat); 20g Protein; 51g Carbohydrate; 94mg Cholesterol; 1311mg Sodium

Sweet and Sour Pork Chops

Serving Size: 6

6 pork loin chops, 3/4 inch thick
1/2 c. pineapple juice, no sugar added
1/2 c. ketchup
2 tbsps. maltitol, honey flavored
2 tbsps. white wine vinegar
1 1/2 tsps. Dijon mustard
1/4 tsp. salt
4 tsps. cornstarch
2 tbsps. water

Preheat oven to 350°F. Place pork chops in a 13 x 9 x 2-inch baking dish. In a bowl, combine pineapple juice, ketchup, maltitol, vinegar, mustard and salt. Pour over the chops. Cover tightly and bake at 350°F for 30 minutes, uncover and bake 30 minutes longer or until meat is tender. Remove chops from pan to a serving platter and keep warm. Strain pan juices into a saucepan. Combine cornstarch and water, stir until cornstarch is completely dissolved; add to pan juices. Cook and stir until thickened and bubbly; cook and stir 2 minutes longer. Pour sauce over chops and serve immediately.

Per serving: 227 Calories; 8g Fat (29% calories from fat); 26g Protein; 14g Carbohydrate; 62mg Cholesterol; 401mg Sodium

Apricot-Baked Chicken

Serving Size: 6

6 boned and skinned chicken breast halves
1 c. apricot nectar, no sugar added
1/2 tsp. ground allspice
1/8 tsp. ground ginger
1/4 tsp. fresh ground black pepper
1/4 tsp. salt
1/3 c. apricot preserves, all fruit (no sugar)
3 tbsps. pecans, toasted

Place the chicken in an oven proof pan large enough that the chicken will not be overlapping. Combine the next 5 ingredients and pour over the chicken, turning the chicken to get the marinade over all parts. Cover tightly and refrigerate overnight or at least 8 hours. Remove from refrigerator and let stand for 30 minutes. Cover tightly with foil and bake in preheated 350°F oven for 30 minutes. Uncover, drain and discard liquid from chicken, and keep warm. Heat apricot preserves and brush over chicken. Bake, uncovered, 20-30 minutes longer, basting with preserves another 2 times. Remove to serving platter and sprinkle with toasted pecans.

Per serving: 176 Calories; 2g Fat (12% calories from fat); 21g Protein; 18g Carbohydrate; 51mg Cholesterol; 155mg Sodium

Chicken and Apples Over Fettucini

Serving Size: 4

4 boneless skinless chicken breast halves, cut into fourths
1 tbsp. canola oil
1 large onion, chopped
1 garlic clove, minced
1/4 c. dry white wine
1 c. apple juice, no sugar added
1 tbsp. fresh ginger root, minced
1 c. low-fat sour cream
1 tbsp. cornstarch
2 Granny Smith apples, cored and chopped
salt and pepper to taste
8 oz. cholesterol-free fettucini or noodles

Remove as much fat as you can from the chicken. Cut chicken and sprinkle them lightly with salt and pepper. Heat oil in skillet large enough to hold chicken pieces in a single layer. Brown chicken on all sides over medium heat; remove and set aside. Chicken should be done at this point since it is cut into small pieces. Saute onion in same pan until onion is soft and translucent. Add garlic, cook one minute, then wine, apple juice and ginger; cook over medium heat until liquid is reduced to 1 cup. Stir cornstarch into sour cream; add to pan with apples and chicken then season to taste. Simmer for about 5 minutes only. While chicken is cooking, prepare pasta or noodles according to instructions on package. Serve chicken and sauce over noodles.

Per serving: 462 Calories; 10g Fat (19% calories from fat); 31g Protein; 60g Carbohydrate; 63mg Cholesterol; 145mg Sodium

Chicken Cacciatore

Serving Size: 6

2 tbsps. olive oil
1 chicken whole, no skin, cut in 8 pieces
1 quart tomatoes, chopped
3 garlic cloves, minced
1/2 tsp. basil
1/2 tsp. oregano
1/2 c. red wine
salt and pepper to taste

Remove skin from chicken. Use a large, heavy pot to saute the onions and garlic in the olive oil. Add the cut-up chicken and brown on all sides. Add remaining ingredients and simmer, covered, for 30 minutes or more until juices run clear from chicken.

Per serving: 254 Calories; 10.9g Fat (40.7% calories from fat); 26.5g Protein; 9.4g Carbohydrate; 78mg Cholesterol; 89mg Sodium

Chicken Dijon

Serving Size: 8

4 oz. plain yogurt
1/4 c. Dijon mustard
8 3 oz. skinless boneless chicken breast halves
1/2 c. soft bread crumbs
 Nonstick cooking spray

Combine yogurt and mustard. Mix well. Coat chicken breasts with yogurt mixture and dredge in bread crumbs. In a 12 x 8 x 2 inch baking dish coated with nonstick cooking spray, arrange chicken. Cover, bake at 400°F for 30 minutes. Increase temperature to 450°F. Bake, uncovered for 15 more minutes or until chicken is done and coating is brown.

Per serving: 119 Calories; 2g Fat (16% calories from fat); 21g Protein; 3g Carbohydrate; 53mg Cholesterol; 172mg Sodium

Chicken Divan

Serving Size: 8

8 2 1/2 oz. skinned and boned chicken breast halves
1 10 oz. frozen broccoli, chopped
Nonstick cooking spray
1/4 can cream of chicken soup, undiluted
1/4 can cream of potato soup, undiluted
1/2 c. skim milk
1 1/2 tsps. lemon juice
2 tbsps. grated Parmesan cheese

In large saucepan, cover chicken with water; cover and bring to boil. Reduce heat and simmer 20 minutes or until chicken is done. Drain. Chop into bite size piece; set aside. Cook broccoli according to directions on package; omitting any salt or fat; drain well. In 2 quart baking or casserole dish coated with cooking spray, place broccoli and top with chicken. In separate bowl, combine soups, milk, and lemon juice; stir to blend. Pour over chicken and broccoli. Sprinkle with Parmesan cheese. Bake at 350°F for 25 minutes or until heated thoroughly.

Per serving: 125 Calories; 2g Fat (15% calories from fat); 23g Protein; 3g Carbohydrate; 53mg Cholesterol; 165mg Sodium

Chicken Fajitas

Serving Size: 4

1 lb. boned and skinned chicken breasts
1 tsp. chili powder
1/4 tsp. pepper
2 cloves garlic, minced
1 medium onion, sliced
chopped fresh cilantro

Spicy Sour Cream
1/2 c. low-fat sour cream
2 tsps. serrano peppers, seeded and chopped

2 tbsps. lime juice
2 tsps. vegetable oil
1/4 tsp. salt
1/2 tsp. ground cumin
8 flour tortillas
1 medium bell pepper, sliced

2 tbsps. lime juice
1/4 tsp. ground cumin

To prepare spicy sour cream, combine all ingredients and chill for at least on hour to blend flavors. Trim fat from chicken breasts, and cut into 1/4 inch slices. Mix lime juice, oil, chili powder, salt, pepper, cumin and garlic in a plastic zip top bag or glass container. Add chicken and toss so that chicken is evenly coated with marinade. Cover and refrigerate at least four hours, but no longer than 12 hours, turning the chicken occasionally. Heat a 10 inch skillet over high heat, then add chicken and cook, stirring constantly for 3 minutes. Add onion and bell pepper and cook for 4 minutes longer. For each serving, place some of the chicken mixture and one tablespoon of the sour cream sauce into a warmed tortilla. Sprinkle with cilantro and fold up tortilla, and enjoy!

Per serving: 440 Calories; 10g Fat (22% calories from fat); 35g Protein; 50g Carbohydrate; 72mg Cholesterol; 586mg Sodium

Chicken Garlic Sticks

Serving Size: 12

2 lbs. skinless boneless chicken breasts, cut into 1" pieces
2 garlic cloves
1/2 c. olive oil
1/4 tsp. hot sauce
1 c. seasoned bread crumbs
3/4 c. Parmesan cheese
1 tsp. pepper

Puree the garlic in the olive oil and hot sauce. Set aside. Combine bread crumbs, cheese and pepper. Set aside. Roll chicken in pureed garlic and then in bread crumbs. Place chicken on cookie sheet that has been prepared with nonstick cooking spray. Bake at 350°F for 30 minutes or until golden and done.

Per serving: 224 Calories; 12g Fat (48% calories from fat); 21g Protein; 7g Carbohydrate; 48mg Cholesterol; 408mg Sodium

Chicken Pomodoro

Serving Size: 4

2 tsps. olive oil
1/2 c. onion, finely chopped
2 cloves garlic, minced
2 1/2 c. chopped tomatoes
2 c. cooked chicken breast halves, cubed
1/4 c. chopped fresh basil
1/2 tsp. salt

Heat oil in a 10 inch skillet over medium high heat. Saute onion about seven minutes or until it is soft. Add garlic and cook for one minute. Add remaining ingredients except basil and reduce heat to medium. Cook for about five minutes, stirring occasionally. until the mixture is hot and the tomatoes are soft. Remove from heat then stir in basil. Serve over your choice of pasta.

Notes: Garlic should only be cooked briefly, just long enough to release the aroma. Cooking it longer can lead to a burnt garlic flavor.

Per serving: 250 Calories; 10g Fat (37% calories from fat); 30g Protein; 9g Carbohydrate; 80mg Cholesterol; 349mg Sodium

Chicken Roasted with Rosemary and Garlic

Serving Size: 6

5 cloves garlic, peeled and halved
1 1/2 tbsps. extra virgin olive oil
3 lbs. roasting chicken, skinless and quartered
2 tbsps. fresh rosemary leaves, minced
1/2 c. white wine

Preheat oven to 350°F. In a 10 inch skillet that is oven-proof, heat oil and garlic over medium high heat. After a couple of minutes, add chicken to the pan and brown lightly on each side. Add rosemary.

Cover skillet and place in the oven. Bake about 45 minutes, or until the juices run clear from the thigh. Remove chicken from pan and set aside, keeping it warm. Put the skillet back on the stove over medium high heat and add the wine. Scrape off any brown pieces that are on the bottom of the pan while stirring. Cook sauce for 3 minutes, strain, then pour it over the chicken and serve.

Per serving: 211 Calories; 7g Fat (35% calories from fat); 30g Protein; 1g Carbohydrate; 96mg Cholesterol; 112mg Sodium

Chicken with Pesto

Serving Size: 4

Pesto Sauce:

1/4 c. chicken broth	2 tbsps. olive oil
1/4 c. grated Parmesan cheese	1 tbsp. pine nuts or pecans
2 cloves garlic	1 c. basil leaves, firmly packed

Chicken & Fettucine

6 oz. fettucine, uncooked	1 1/2 tsps. olive oil
1/2 c. red bell pepper, chopped	1/2 c. chopped onion
1 c. asparagus spears, cut in 1 inch pieces	1 1/2 c. cooked chicken breast halves, cubed
1 c. fresh mushrooms, sliced	

To prepare pesto, combine all ingredients in a food processor and process until almost smooth. Cook fettucine according to package directions and drain, set aside and keep warm. Heat oil in a 10 inch skillet over high heat, add asparagus, mushrooms, red bell pepper, and onion. Stir while it is cooking about four minutes, then reduce heat. Stir in chicken and heat thoroughly. Remove form heat then stir in pesto the fettucine. Toss with forks to evenly distribute pesto and vegetables.

Notes: Pesto sauce should never be heated because it discolors the basil leaves. If you have any leftover pesto, refrigerate it, and when you have to use it again, let it sit at room temperature to warm a little before using it.

Per serving: 450 Calories; 18g Fat (36% calories from fat); 32g Protein; 39g Carbohydrate; 65mg Cholesterol; 273mg Sodium

Curried Chicken

Serving Size: 8

1 large apple, unpeeled and chopped
1/4 c. green onion, sliced
1 tbsp. curry powder
1 tbsp. water
1 c. skim milk
2 tbsps. fresh parsley, minced
2 c. chicken breasts without skin, cooked and chopped
1/2 c. plain low-fat yogurt

Combine apple, green onions, curry powder and water in medium saucepan. Cover and cook over medium heat until onions are tender. Add water, milk and parsley, stir until mixed well. Add chicken, simmer 10 minutes. Reduce to low and stir in yogurt. Cook, stirring gently until thoroughly heated.
Notes: Serve over hot rice that has been prepared without salt or fat.

Per serving: 85 Calories; 1g Fat (11% calories from fat); 13g Protein; 6g Carbohydrate; 29mg Cholesterol; 58mg Sodium

Grilled Marinated Chicken

Serving Size: 6

3 tbsps. lemon juice
3 tbsps. vinegar
2 tbsps. low-fat mayonnaise
1/4 c. maltitol plus 2 tbsps.
1/2 tsp. salt, optional
1/2 tsp. pepper
6 2 1/2 oz. skinless boneless chicken breast halves

Combine all ingredients except chicken, mix well. Place chicken in shallow container and cover with marinade. Cover container and refrigerate at least 1 hour. Remove chicken from marinade. Grill chicken 45 minutes or until done.

Notes: This recipe was prepared cooking over hot coals. Adjust time accordingly for grilling inside.

Per serving: 136 Calories; 2g Fat (16% calories from fat); 20g Protein; 10g Carbohydrate; 53mg Cholesterol; 259mg Sodium

Heart Healthy Oriental Chicken and Vegetables

Serving Size: 4

4 boned and skinned chicken breasts, cubed
2 garlic cloves, minced
1 can baby corn
1 onion, minced
1 red pepper, julienned
1 green bell pepper, julienned
1 tbsp. cornstarch
4 tbsps. soy sauce, low sodium
8 oz. pineapple chunks, in juice
2 tbsps. vinegar
3 tbsps. brown sugar replacement
1/2 tsp. ground ginger
2 c. cooked rice

Heat a heavy skillet; add 1 tablespoon oil. Saute the peppers, garlic and onion until onion is limp. Remove from skillet and keep warm. Add 1 tablespoon oil to skillet and cook chicken cubes until all turn white and are cooked through. Mix cornstarch with soy sauce and some of the pineapple juice in a small bowl. Combine the chicken with the onion mixture. Add the pineapple chunks and juice along with the baby corn, brown sugar replacement substitute, vinegar and ground or freshly grated ginger. Heat to boiling, then add the cornstarch mixture. Stir constantly until sauce is thickened and heated through. Serve immediately over hot cooked white rice.

Per serving: 394 Calories; 3g Fat (6% calories from fat); 44g Protein; 47g Carbohydrate; 96mg Cholesterol; 717mg Sodium

Lemon-Pineapple Chicken

Serving Size: 6

20 oz. pineapple chunks in juice, no sugar added
2 garlic cloves, minced
1 tbsp. cornstarch
1 tsp. Worcestershire sauce
2 tsps. Dijon mustard
1/4 tsp. dried rosemary, ground
1 tsp. salt
1 lemon, thinly sliced
6 chicken breast halves without skin

Preheat oven to 350°F. Drain pineapple; combine the juice with garlic, cornstarch, Worcestershire sauce, mustard and rosemary. Set aside. Arrange chicken in shallow pan, bone side down. Sprinkle with salt. Broil until browned. Stir the sauce and pour over the chicken. Bake at 350°F for about 25 minutes, depending on thickness of chicken. Arrange pineapple and thin lemon slices around chicken, baste with the sauce in pan and continue baking 5 minutes longer.

Per serving: 192 Calories; 2g Fat (7% calories from fat); 27g Protein; 19g Carbohydrate; 65mg Cholesterol; 459mg Sodium

Orange Chicken Stir-Fry

Serving Size: 4

4 each chicken breasts without skin, boneless	1 tsp. cornstarch
1 tbsp. soy sauce	2 cloves garlic, minced
1/2 c. orange juice	1/2 tsp. ground ginger
4 tsps. sesame oil	2 tsps. cornstarch
1/2 c. carrot, coarsely shredded	3 c. fresh mushrooms, sliced
4 c. cooked rice	1/2 c. zucchini, coarsely shredded

Trim fat from chicken breast halves and cut into 1/4 inch strips. Combine soy sauce, one teaspoon cornstarch, ginger, and garlic in a bowl or plastic bag and add chicken. Toss the chicken to make sure it is completely covered by the marinade. Refrigerate for an hour. Mix the orange juice, and 2 teaspoons cornstarch until the cornstarch is completely dissolved. Heat 2 teaspoons sesame oil in a 10 inch skillet over high heat then add chicken mixture. Stir fry the chicken until it turns white, then remove it from the skillet. Add the remaining sesame oil to the skillet, then add mushrooms, carrot and zucchini, stir fry about 3 minutes, then stir in chicken and orange juice mixture. Heat until mixture boils, then boil one minute, stirring constantly. Serve over hot rice.

Notes: Another vegetable oil can be substituted for sesame oil, but the sesame oil adds lots of flavor to dishes low in fat. Toasted sesame oil is equally delicious, although harder to find.

Per serving: 584 Calories; 8g Fat (13% calories from fat); 59g Protein; 64g Carbohydrate; 130mg Cholesterol; 419mg Sodium

Paella

Serving Size: 8

8 boned and skinned chicken breast halves, cut into pieces	2 tbsps. olive oil
2 garlic cloves	1/2 c. chopped onions
2 c. rice	1 tsp. olive oil
4 c. nonfat chicken broth	1 pinch saffron
1 lb. cooked shrimp	2 c. green peas
1 Italian sausage, sliced	1 c. extra lean ham, chopped
	24 cherrystone clams in shells

Prepare all ingredients before beginning assembly. Scrub clams well. Cook shrimp or buy precooked. Slice sausage and chop the ham. Cut chicken into serving sized pieces. Cook green peas until barely tender. Chop onions and minced garlic. Use a very heavy skillet to heat the olive oil. Add cut-up skinned chicken pieces. Brown well on all sides then add 1/2 cup water. Cover tightly and cook until chicken is tender, about 30-35 minutes. Remove chicken from pan and set aside. Add the onion and garlic to the pan juices; cook slowly for 5 minutes. In a medium saucepan, heat oil then add uncooked rice and a pinch of saffron. Stir over low heat for 5 minutes. Add 4 cups broth. Bring to a boil, cover, and cook on low heat for 17-18 minutes. Stir the rice mixture into the pan with the onions and garlic. Add green peas and blend well. Use a 4-quart casserole or a paella pan to finish preparations. Layer the rice, chicken, shrimp, ham and sausage in pan. Bury some of the clams partially into the mixture. Place rest of clams on top. Bake at 350°F until paella is heated through and clams are open. Discard any clams that do not open.

Per serving: 501 Calories; 12g Fat (23% calories from fat); 50g Protein; 45g Carbohydrate; 193mg Cholesterol; 739mg Sodium

Pasta with Chicken and Peas

Serving Size: 4

4 c. pasta shells, small
2 c. boned and skinned chicken breasts, cooked and chopped
2 tbsps. shallots, minced
2 tsps. olive oil
1/2 c. green peas
3 cloves minced garlic
1 tsp. dried basil
1/2 tsp. dried thyme
3 tbsps. chopped fresh parsley
1/4 c. red bell pepper, minced
1/2 c. grated Parmesan cheese

Preheat oven to 400°F. Cook pasta in a large pot, just until almost done. Drain and rinse in cold water then set aside. In a 10 inch skillet over medium high heat, saute the chicken and shallots in olive oil for 2 minutes, then add the peas, garlic, herbs and bell pepper. Cook a couple minutes more then pour it all into a large baking dish and combine it with the pasta shells and Parmesan cheese. Bake for 20 minutes.

Per serving: 622 Calories; 9g Fat (14% calories from fat); 47g Protein; 84g Carbohydrate; 79mg Cholesterol; 322mg Sodium

Rosemary and Lemon Chicken

Serving Size: 4

1 1/2 c. fresh mushrooms, sliced
2 cloves garlic, minced
1 tbsp. extra virgin olive oil
4 each boned and skinned chicken breast halves
2 tbsps. all-purpose flour
1/4 tsp. dried rosemary, ground
1/4 c. fresh lemon juice
1/4 c. chicken broth
2 tbsps. fresh parsley, minced
1/4 tsp. black pepper

In a 10 inch skillet, saute mushrooms in oil over medium heat for five minutes. Add garlic and saute one minute more. Remove from pan. Combine flour and rosemary and dust chicken with this mixture. Add chicken to skillet and brown on both sides. Add lemon juice and broth to chicken and stir, scraping up any browned bits from the bottom of the pan. Return mushrooms to the pan, cover and simmer for 15 minutes. Add parsley and pepper and serve.

Per serving: 157 Calories; 5g Fat (28% calories from fat); 22g Protein; 6g Carbohydrate; 51mg Cholesterol; 158mg Sodium

Salsa Baked Chicken

Serving Size: 4

4 each boned and skinned chicken breasts
1 c. salsa
1 tbsp. lime juice
2 tbsps. fresh cilantro, chopped

Preheat oven to 400°F. Place chicken breast halves in a baking dish big enough so that they all fit single layer. Combine salsa, lime juice and cilantro and pour over chicken. Bake chicken for 20-25 minutes.

Per serving: 202 Calories; 3g Fat (14% calories from fat); 39g Protein; 4g Carbohydrate; 96mg Cholesterol; 544mg Sodium

Spicy Indian Chicken

Serving Size: 4

1 tsp. ground turmeric
1 tsp. coriander
1/8 tsp. chili powder
3 tbsps. butter or margarine
2 onions, chopped fine
2 tomatoes, chopped
1 celery stalks, chopped fine
3 parsley sprigs, minced
1/3 c. seedless raisins
1 1/2 tsps. lemon juice

1 tsp. curry powder
1/2 tsp. ground ginger
black pepper to taste
4 boneless skinless chicken breast halves, cubed
2 green bell peppers, chopped fine
2 garlic cloves, minced
1 tbsp. dry sherry

Heat two tablespoons butter in a large skillet. Place first six ingredients (all the spices) in skillet and brown for 1 minute over high heat. Place chicken in skillet with browned spices; stir to coat well, then brown 1 minute longer or until chicken has turned white on the inside. Remove from pan and set aside. Add remaining butter to pan and saute onions over high heat until soft. Add remaining ingredients, including browned chicken, and cook over medium heat until celery is tender but still slightly crisp. Vegetables will give off some juiciness as they cook.

Per serving: 279 Calories; 10g Fat (33% calories from fat); 23g Protein; 24g Carbohydrate; 74mg Cholesterol; 167mg Sodium

Spicy Oven Fried Drumsticks

Serving Size: 4

8 chicken drumstick, no skin
1/3 c. all-purpose flour
1/3 c. yellow cornmeal
1/4 tsp. dried oregano
1 tsp. ground cumin
1/2 tsp. chili powder
1/4 tsp. salt
1 pinch ground cloves
1/3 c. low-fat buttermilk
1/4 tsp. hot sauce
1 tbsp. vegetable oil

Heat oven to 400 °F. Spray 9 X 13 inch pan with nonstick Nonstick cooking spray. Remove skin and fat from chicken drumsticks. Mix remaining ingredients except buttermilk and hot sauce. In a large plastic bag. Combine buttermilk and hot sauce in a bowl. Dip each chicken drumstick in the buttermilk mixture, then place in the bag of flour mixture and shake until completely coated. Repeat this with each drumstick and place them in the prepared pan. Spray or drizzle with the vegetable oil and bake uncovered for 40 to 45 minutes or until done.

Per serving: 234 Calories; 7.8g Fat (30.9% calories from fat); 20.9g Protein; 18.6g Carbohydrate; 59mg Cholesterol; 220mg Sodium

Turkey and Spinach Enchiladas

Serving Size: 6

1 lb. ground turkey

1 1/2 c. picante sauce

1 1/2 tsps. ground cumin

1 tsp. chili powder

10 oz. frozen chopped spinach, thawed and drained

8 oz. low-fat cream cheese, cubed

12 corn tortillas

14 1/2 oz. canned tomatoes, diced

1 c. low-fat cheddar cheese

In a 10 inch skillet over medium high heat, combine turkey, cumin, and chili powder and cook until turkey is no longer pink, then pour off the fat. Add one cup of the picante sauce, and spinach, and heat until boiling. Reduce heat to low and cook five minutes. Add cream cheese and stir until melted.

Spread about 1/3 cup of meat mixture down the center of each tortilla, roll the tortilla up and place seam side down on in a 9X13 ovenproof baking dish. Repeat until all of mixture is used.

Combine tomatoes and remaining picante sauce. Spoon over enchiladas, cover and bake at 350°F for 30 minutes. Uncover, top with cheese and bake five minutes more or until cheese has melted. Serve piping hot.

Per serving: 415 Calories; 19g Fat (40% calories from fat); 29g Protein; 35g Carbohydrate; 90mg Cholesterol; 1153mg Sodium

Vegetables

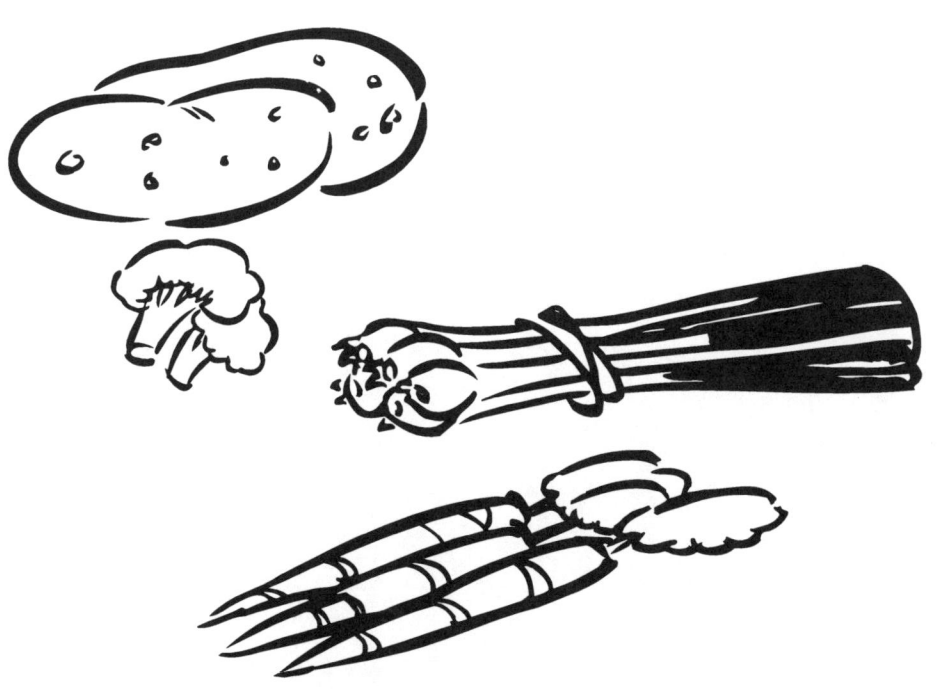

Asparagus Torta

Serving Size: 4

1/2 tbsp. butter
1 medium onion, minced
2 green onions, minced
1/4 tsp. dried sage
1 tbsp. fresh chives, minced
3/4 c. liquid egg substitute, plus 2 tbsps.
1/2 c. grated Parmesan cheese
1 c. part-skim ricotta cheese
1 1/2 c. asparagus tips, cooked
 salt and pepper to taste

Preheat oven to 450°F. In a 6 inch ovenproof skillet, melt the butter over medium heat and saute both onions until they are soft, about 6 minutes. While the onions are cooking, combine herbs, egg substitute, Parmesan and ricotta cheese and beat until smooth. Add the asparagus to the skillet and stir to mix with the onions. Pour the egg and cheese mixture on top. Put the skillet in the oven and bake until a knife inserted in the center comes out clean, about 35 minutes. Serve at any temperature.

Per serving: 249 Calories; 12g Fat (43% calories from fat); 22g Protein; 15g Carbohydrate; 33mg Cholesterol; 415mg Sodium

Baked Acorn Squash

Serving Size: 4

1 medium acorn squash, quartered
1 tbsp. butter
1/4 c. brown sugar replacement
1/4 tsp. salt
1 dash pepper

Preheat the oven to 350°F. After the squash has been quartered, scrape out all the seeds and place then on a baking sheet. Melt the butter and combine it with the Sugar Twin, salt, and pepper. Brush the glaze onto the squash, reserving a little of the glaze for later. Bake squash, uncovered, for about 30 minutes, or until the squash is easily pierced with a fork. Remove squash from the oven and baste with additional glaze. Serve hot.

Notes: It is not necessary to peel acorn squash before cooking it (it's a pain in the neck). Just eat it by scraping the cooked squash off of the skin.

Per serving: 52 Calories; 3g Fat (46% calories from fat); 1g Protein; 7g Carbohydrate; 8mg Cholesterol; 164mg Sodium

Balsamic Marinated Vegetables

Serving Size: 6

4 c. mixed vegetables
2/3 c. extra virgin olive oil
1/3 c. white wine
1/4 c. balsamic vinegar
1/2 c. chopped onions
4 garlic cloves, minced
1/2 tsp. basil
1/4 tsp. thyme
1/8 tsp. cayenne pepper
 black pepper to taste
1/4 c. fresh parsley, finely chopped

Ideas for vegetables: green beans, broccoli florets, cauliflower, red and green bell peppers, whole baby carrots, zucchini, celery, or artichoke hearts.

Combine all ingredients except 2 teaspoons parsley in a large, heavy pot. Add enough water to cover vegetables. Cover and cook over medium heat until vegetables are just tender but still crisp, about 10-12 minutes. Remove from heat, remove cover, and let vegetables cool in the pot. When cool, transfer to serving dish. Cover; chill to allow flavors to blend. Bring to room temperature to serve; top with remaining parsley.

Per serving: 291 Calories; 24g Fat (76% calories from fat); 3g Protein; 14g Carbohydrate; 0mg Cholesterol; 370mg Sodium

Boiled Parslied New Potatoes

Serving Size: 5

1 lb. red potatoes, small
2 tbsps. butter
1 1/2 tbsps. chopped fresh parsley
1/2 tsp. salt
1/4 tsp. pepper

Bring a large pot of water to boil. Add potatoes and cook until tender, about 10-20 minutes, depending on size. Drain the potatoes and add the butter, stirring gently until it melts. Add the parsley, salt and pepper, mix gently and serve.

Per serving: 95 Calories; 5g Fat (43% calories from fat); 2g Protein; 12g Carbohydrate; 12mg Cholesterol; 264mg Sodium

Broccoli with Pearl Onions Casserole

Serving Size: 8

20 oz. frozen broccoli florets
4 tbsps. butter
1/4 tsp. salt
1 c. skim milk, cold
1/4 tsp. dried thyme
1 c. soft breadcrumbs

1 1/2 c. frozen pearl onions
2 tbsps. flour
1 dash pepper
3 oz. nonfat cream cheese, cut into bits
1/4 c. grated Parmesan cheese

Preheat the oven to 350°F. Cook broccoli and anions according to package directions, drain both and set aside. In a medium skillet, melt half the butter over medium heat. Add flour and stir until a paste forms. Keep stirring the paste for three minutes, you might want to reduce the heat a little if the mixture starts to brown too much. Whisk in the milk, and add the seasonings, stirring until all lumps are gone. Increase the heat to medium high and stir constantly until very thick and bubbly. Reduce the heat to medium, and stir in the cream cheese until well blended. Add the broccoli and onions to the sauce mixture and mix until everything is well coated. Spray a 1 1/2 quart casserole dish with nonstick cooking spray and pour in vegetables and sauce. Bake uncovered for 20 minutes. While casserole is cooking, melt the remaining butter and toss it with the breadcrumbs and cheese. Sprinkle this over the casserole and bake for 40 more minutes.

Notes: A heated mixture of even parts fat (such as oil or butter) and flour is called a "roux". The reason to keep cooking the roux after it has formed a paste is to cook out the starchy flavor of the flour.

Per serving: 137 Calories; 7g Fat (46% calories from fat); 7g Protein; 12g Carbohydrate; 20mg Cholesterol; 306mg Sodium

Broiled Tomatoes with Horseradish

Serving Size: 4

2 large tomatoes
2 tbsps. seasoned bread crumbs
2 tbsps. horseradish
1 tbsp. lemon juice
1/8 tsp. salt
1/4 tsp. paprika
2 tsps. fresh parsley
4 tbsps. grated Parmesan cheese

Set oven to broil. Cut tomatoes in half, crosswise. Combine breadcrumbs, horseradish, lemon juice, salt and paprika. Spread mixture over tomatoes halves. Sprinkle with chopped parsley and the cheese. Place in a broiler pan; broil 3 inches from heat 3-5 minutes until heated through. Serve immediately.

Per serving: 65 Calories; 2g Fat (28% calories from fat); 4g Protein; 8g Carbohydrate; 5mg Cholesterol; 298mg Sodium

Buttermilk Mashed Potatoes

Serving Size: 6

2 lbs. potatoes, peeled and quartered
1/2 c. low-fat buttermilk
2 tbsps. minced fresh chives
1 tbsp. butter
 salt and pepper to taste

Place potatoes in boiling water and cook until easily cut with a fork, about 15-20 minutes, drain. In a bowl, combine potatoes, buttermilk, and butter. Mash with a potato masher until all large lumps are gone. Stir in chives and season to taste with salt and pepper. Serve hot.

Notes: Whipping potatoes in an electric mixer for too long makes potatoes gluey, try whipping them not as long or using a potato masher for fluffier potatoes.

Per serving: 115 Calories; 2g Fat (17% calories from fat); 3g Protein; 21g Carbohydrate; 6mg Cholesterol; 47mg Sodium

Cabbage Casserole

Serving Size: 4

1 c. skim milk
1 egg beaten
1/4 tsp. salt
1 c. cabbage, grated
1/4 c. American cheese, low-fat and shredded
Nonstick cooking spray

Combine milk, egg and salt in medium bowl. Mix well. Fold in cabbage and cheese. Pour in 1 quart casserole dish that has been prepared with nonstick cooking spray. Bake at 400°F for 30 minutes or until done.

Per serving: 66 Calories; 3g Fat (46% calories from fat); 5g Protein; 4g Carbohydrate; 53mg Cholesterol; 227mg Sodium

Chili Topped Potatoes

Serving Size: 6

1 lb. extra lean ground beef
1 tbsp. chili powder
1 c. salsa
6 russet potatoes, baked and hot
2/3 c. nonfat cheddar cheese, grated
1/4 c. green onions, minced

In a 10 inch skillet over medium high heat, cook beef and chili powder until beef is browned, stirring frequently to separate meat. Pour off fat. Add salsa, reduce heat to low and simmer 3 minutes. Spoon some of the meat mixture into each potato and garnish with cheese and minced green onion.

Per serving: 424 Calories; 14g Fat (29% calories from fat); 24g Protein; 52g Carbohydrate; 54mg Cholesterol; 459mg Sodium

Creamy Green Beans

Serving Size: 6

1 1/2 lbs. green beans, fresh
8 oz. water chestnuts, canned and drained
1/4 c. green onion sliced
1/2 c. low-fat cream cheese
1/2 tsp. white wine vinegar
 salt and pepper to taste

Bring a large pot of water to boiling. Once pot is boiling, drop in green beans and cook for 8 minutes - this should cook the beans to a perfect tenderness without losing their bright green color. While the beans are coking, combine remaining ingredients in a saucepan over low heat until cheese is melted and sauce is warm. Drain green beans and toss with sauce.

Per serving: 95 Calories; 3g Fat (31% calories from fat); 4g Protein; 13g Carbohydrate; 11mg Cholesterol; 141mg Sodium

Duo of Grilled Squash

Serving Size: 4

1 clove garlic, minced
2 tsps. extra virgin olive oil
1 tsp. dried whole basil
1/2 tsp. dried whole oregano
1/4 tsp. lemon pepper
1/4 tsp. salt
2 medium zucchini
2 medium yellow squash

Cut all of the squash in half lengthwise, set aside. Combine garlic, olive oil, and seasonings and heat in a small sauce pan over low heat until warm and aromatic. Brush cut surfaces of the squash with half of the garlic mixture. Place vegetables on a preheated grill, cut side down, and grill for 4 minutes. Turn vegetables over and brush with remaining garlic mixture. Cook for 4 more minutes or until done. Serve as a side dish or as a snack dipped in tomato sauce.

Per serving: 44 Calories; 3g Fat (46% calories from fat); 2g Protein; 5g Carbohydrate; 0mg Cholesterol; 158mg Sodium

Florentine Frittata

Serving Size: 4

2 tsps. extra virgin olive oil
1 tbsp. minced green onion
3/4 c. liquid egg substitute
1/2 c. grated Parmesan cheese
1/2 tsp. dried whole basil
1/8 tsp. black pepper
1 c. cooked spinach, drained and chopped

Set oven to broil. Heat the olive oil in an 8-inch skillet over medium heat. Add the onion and cook for 3 minutes. Combine the egg substitute with 1/3 cup of the cheese, basil, and spinach, and mix with a spoon, careful not to incorporate much air into the mixture. Pour the egg mixture into the skillet and stir once or twice just to mix in the onions. Cook over very low heat until the edges are lightly browned. Remove from heat and sprinkle the remaining cheese on top and place the skillet under the broiler until the cheese is lightly browned. To serve, cut into wedges. This dish is good hot or cold.

Per serving: 128 Calories; 8g Fat (54% calories from fat); 12g Protein; 3g Carbohydrate; 10mg Cholesterol; 350mg Sodium

Fresh Glazed Beets

Serving Size: 5

1 lb. fresh beets
2 tbsps. butter
1 1/2 tsps. fresh lemon juice
2 tbsps. maltitol-sweetened maple syrup
 salt and pepper to taste

Wash beets and trim the tops so that they are 2 inches long. In a large pot, boil the beets in their skins until they are tender (easily pierced all the way through with a knife). Drain the beets and let them cool until easily handled. Peel the beets and cut them into thin slices. Melt the butter in a 10 inch skillet then add the lemon juice, Country Syrup and beets. Cook the beets over high heat until liquids in the pan are a thick glaze, then season to taste.

Per serving: 79 Calories; 5g Fat (49% calories from fat); 1g Protein; 10g Carbohydrate; 12mg Cholesterol; 95mg Sodium

Gingered Carrots

Serving Size: 6

2 c. carrots sliced 1/4 inch thick
2 tsps. melted butter
1 c. fresh orange juice
1/2 tsp. ground ginger
1/2 c. chicken stock, cold
1 tsp. cornstarch
 salt and pepper to taste

Combine carrots, butter and orange juice in a skillet over medium high heat and bring to a boil. Reduce heat, cover, and simmer 5-8 minutes or until carrots are fork tender. Combine cornstarch, chicken stock and ginger in a cup and stir until cornstarch is dissolved. Add mixture to carrots while stirring constantly and bring to a boil. Allow mixture to boil one minute then remove from heat and season to taste.

Notes: When using cornstarch, make sure to dissolve it in a cold liquid before adding it to something hot. Cornstarch added alone to hot ingredients will clump up and not thicken the way you want it to.

Per serving: 48 Calories; 1g Fat (27% calories from fat); 1g Protein; 8g Carbohydrate; 3mg Cholesterol; 204mg Sodium

Green Beans with Toasted Pecans

Serving Size: 4

3/4 lb. green beans, split lengthwise
3 tbsps. chicken stock, hot
2 tsps. minced shallots
1 tsp. minced garlic
1 1/2 tsps. melted butter
3 tbsps. chopped pecans toasted (see note)
2 tsps. chopped fresh chives

Place the green beans in a pan with the hot stock. Sprinkle over them the remaining ingredients. Cover the skillet and cook over medium high heat for 3 minutes or until the beans are tender.
Notes: To toast pecans, place them on a baking sheet in a 350°F oven for about 5-8 minutes or until they are very aromatic.

Per serving: 57 Calories; 3g Fat (48% calories from fat); 2g Protein; 6g Carbohydrate; 4mg Cholesterol; 120mg Sodium

Grilled Vegetables

Serving Size: 4

6 c. eggplant, peeled and cubed
1 large green bell pepper, chopped
1 large onion, chopped
1 tbsp. olive oil
1/4 tsp. dried basil
2 medium tomatoes
 salt and pepper to taste

 Peel and cube eggplant to make about 6 cups. Mix with the chopped green pepper and chopped onion. Cut 3 pieces of heavy foil about 12 x 18 inches. Divide the eggplant mixture evenly on foil. Place 1 teaspoon olive oil on mixture; sprinkle with basil, or if preferred use chopped fresh basil. Close foil tightly. Place foil packs on grill 3-4 inches from heat; cook for about 35 minutes. Chop tomato and place on another piece of foil. Close foil and place on grill the last 15 minutes of eggplant cooking time. Remove vegetables from foil; blend together in large bowl. Season to taste with salt and black pepper.

Per serving: 92 Calories; 4g Fat (34% calories from fat); 2g Protein; 15g Carbohydrate; 0mg Cholesterol; 11mg Sodium

Grilled Potatoes

Serving Size: 4

1 lb. red potatoes, quartered
1 medium sweet green peppers, cubed
1 medium onion, sliced
2 tbsps. extra virgin olive oil
1/2 tsp. dried rosemary, ground
2 cloves garlic, minced
1/2 tsp. salt
1/4 tsp. black pepper

Combine potatoes, pepper and onion in a large bowl and set aside. Combine oil, rosemary, and garlic. Toss oil mixture with potato mixture and sprinkle all with salt and pepper. Place veggies in a large square of heavy aluminum foil and seal it shut. Place foil package on the grill over medium to hot coals and cook for 45 minutes turning once, or until vegetables are soft.

Notes: It is best if you use the smaller red bliss potatoes for this recipe.

Per serving: 148 Calories; 7g Fat (41% calories from fat); 2g Protein; 20g Carbohydrate; 0mg Cholesterol; 274mg Sodium

Italian Style Green Beans

Serving Size: 4

1 lb. green beans
2 Roma tomatoes
1/4 c. grated Parmesan cheese
1/4 tsp. salt
1/8 tsp. pepper
1 tbsp. minced fresh basil

Cook green beans in boiling water for 8 minutes if fresh, or according to packages directions if frozen. While beans are cooking, cut tomatoes into fourths, and remove seeds and white part from top. Slice tomatoes into thin strips and set aside. After beans are cooked, combine them with tomatoes and all other ingredients and toss them so that all ingredients are well mixed. Serve hot.

Notes: Fresh Parmesan cheese can be bought in the deli section of the store in whole chunks, and while it is a hassle to grate sometimes, it has a much stronger and richer flavor than the Parmesan bought in a can.

Per serving: 72 Calories; 2g Fat (25% calories from fat); 5g Protein; 10g Carbohydrate; 5mg Cholesterol; 262mg Sodium

Maple Baked Beans

Serving Size: 6

2 c. dried navy beans, rinsed
1 onion, chopped
1 large clove garlic, chopped fine
1/2 lb. Canadian bacon, chopped
8 c. water
1/2 c. maltitol-sweetened maple syrup
1 tsp. dry mustard
1/2 tsp. paprika

In 7 1/2 quart ovenproof heavy kettle, combine beans, onion, garlic, bacon and water. Simmer, covered partially, 1 hour. Add remaining ingredients. Ladle out, reserving 1/2 cup cooking liquid. Bake at 300°F, 1 hour adding liquid as needed to keep from drying out.

Per serving: 343 Calories; 4g Fat (9% calories from fat); 24g Protein; 58g Carbohydrate; 19mg Cholesterol; 558mg Sodium

Marinated Broccoli

Serving Size: 6

2 lbs. fresh broccoli or 20 oz. frozen
1/4 c. extra virgin olive oil
1 clove garlic, crushed
1/2 tsp. salt
1/2 tsp. pepper
2 tbsps. fresh lemon juice

Cook broccoli until crisp tender or use thawed, not cooked, frozen. Place in serving bowl, set aside. Whisk together remaining ingredients. Pour over broccoli and let stand before serving. Serve at room temperature.

Per serving: 124 Calories; 10g Fat (62% calories from fat); 5g Protein; 9g Carbohydrate; 0mg Cholesterol; 219mg Sodium

Mushroom Barley

Serving Size: 6

1 tbsp. butter
4 cloves garlic, minced
1 c. fresh parsley, minced
1 c. shiitake mushrooms, washed and sliced
1 c. uncooked pearl barley, rinsed
2 tbsps. white wine
2 c. chicken stock
 salt and pepper to taste

In a medium saucepan, melt the butter over medium low heat and add garlic and parsley, cooking just to release flavors, about 3 minutes. Add the mushrooms and cook, stirring constantly, until they soften, about three more minutes. Add the barley, wine and broth and turn the heat up to high - bring the mixture to a boil. Lower heat to medium-low and cover, then simmer for 40 minutes. Turn the heat off and let stand for 10 more minutes. Fluff with a fork before serving.

Per serving: 186 Calories; 3g Fat (12% calories from fat); 5g Protein; 36g Carbohydrate; 5mg Cholesterol; 746mg Sodium

Peas with Mint

Serving Size: 8

2 c. green peas, cooked
2 tbsps. butter, melted
1/4 tsp. salt
1/2 c. fresh mint leaves, minced

Combine all ingredients and combine well. This dish is good served hot or chilled.

Per serving: 55 Calories; 3g Fat (48% calories from fat); 2g Protein; 5g Carbohydrate; 8mg Cholesterol; 98mg Sodium

Potato Cheese Casserole

Serving Size: 8

3 c. mashed potatoes, cooked
1 egg, separated
1/2 c. American cheese, low-fat and shredded
1/2 small green pepper, finely chopped
1 tbsp. green onions, finely chopped
1/2 tsp. celery salt
1 egg white
 Nonstick cooking spray
1/2 tsp. paprika

Combine mashed potatoes and egg yolk. Mix well. Add cheese, green pepper, green onions and celery salt. Mix well. Beat 2 egg whites (room temperature) at high speed with electric mixer until soft peaks form. Gently fold egg whites into potato mixture. Spoon into 1 1/2 quart casserole dish that has been prepared with nonstick cooking spray. Sprinkle with paprika. Bake at 375°F for 25 to 30 minutes or until done. Serve immediately.

Per serving: 105 Calories; 4g Fat (32% calories from fat); 5g Protein; 13g Carbohydrate; 31mg Cholesterol; 339mg Sodium

Potato Gratin

Serving Size: 4

2 c. skim milk, plus 2 tbsps.
2 lbs. red potatoes, thinly sliced
2 cloves garlic, minced
1/2 tsp. salt
1/4 tsp. pepper
1 tbsp. cornstarch
1/2 c. Swiss cheese, shredded
1/4 c. grated Parmesan cheese

Preheat oven to 375°F. In a medium saucepan, combine 2 cups of milk, potatoes, garlic and salt and pepper. Bring this to a simmer over medium high heat and cook until the potatoes are tender, about 10 minutes. Using a slotted spoon, transfer the potatoes to a baking dish that has been sprayed with nonstick cooking spray. In a cup, combine the cornstarch and the remaining milk until the cornstarch is dissolved. Whisk the paste into the hot milk that was left from cooking the potatoes in, and cook about 10 minutes over medium high heat or until the mixture simmers. Stir the grated Swiss cheese into the milk mixture until melted, them pour the whole thing over the potatoes. Sprinkle with Parmesan and bake until the cheese is slightly browned, about 15 minutes. Allow to set 10 minutes before serving to let the dish firm up (and to keep from burning your tongue!).

Per serving: 269 Calories; 6g Fat (20% calories from fat); 14g Protein; 40g Carbohydrate; 20mg Cholesterol; 494mg Sodium

Red Potato Casserole

Serving Size: 6

3 lbs. red potatoes, small
1 medium onion, chopped
1 lb. mushrooms, sliced
1/3 cup olive oil
2 cloves garlic, minced
1/8 tsp. dried rosemary ground
1/4 tsp. dried basil
1/4 tsp. dried oregano

Preheat oven to 325°F. Boil potatoes whole until almost done then cut each one in half. Place into a 2 quart baking dish that has been sprayed with nonstick cooking spray (olive oil flavored, if you have some on hand). Place the mushrooms, onion and garlic over the potatoes, then sprinkle the seasonings over the top. Drizzle the olive oil over the top and bake 15-20 minutes or until the potatoes are done.

Per serving: 270 Calories; 13g Fat (40% calories from fat); 5g Protein; 37g Carbohydrate; 0mg Cholesterol; 14mg Sodium

Roasted Corn Relish

Serving Size: 6

6 ears corn
2 tbsps. white wine vinegar
1 red bell pepper, minced
3 green onions, minced
1 poblano peppers, minced
 salt and pepper to taste

To roast corn, preheat oven to 400°F and place corn in the oven without removing any of the husk. Bake until it is very aromatic and the corn is tender, about 15-20 minutes. Remove the corn from the husk and remove all the corn silk from the corn. To scrape the corn from the ear, hold the ear at an angle and take a sharp knife and run it down the length of the corn, scraping off the corn as you go. Combine all the corn with the remaining ingredients and serve at any temperature.

Notes: If poblano peppers are not available in your area, choose a pepper that is mildly hot, or substitute any pepper you like that will give a little "heat" to the dish!

Per serving: 96 Calories; 1g Fat (9% calories from fat); 4g Protein; 22g Carbohydrate; 0mg Cholesterol; 15mg Sodium

Savory Potato Casserole

Serving Size: 8

6 large potatoes, peeled
1/4 c. butter
2 c. nonfat cheddar cheese, shredded
2 c. nonfat sour cream
1/3 c. green onions, chopped
1 tsp. salt
1/4 tsp. black pepper
1 tbsp. chopped fresh parsley

Preheat oven to 350°F. Boil potatoes whole until tender, drain. Place potatoes in the refrigerator until cold, then remove them and grate coarsely. Combine potatoes with remaining ingredients and pour into a 2 quart casserole that has been sprayed with nonstick cooking spray. Bake for 45 minutes.

Per serving: 290 Calories; 6g Fat (18% calories from fat); 18g Protein; 44g Carbohydrate; 30mg Cholesterol; 582mg Sodium

Sesame Broccoli

Serving Size: 6

4 c. broccoli florets
2 tsps. sesame oil
2 tsps. rice vinegar
1 tbsp. sesame seeds, toasted
 salt and pepper to taste

Remove tough stems from broccoli; wash, then cut heads into florets. Steam for 7-8 minutes, or until broccoli is tender but still crisp. Mix sesame oil with vinegar in a serving bowl. Add steamed broccoli and mix gently to coat. Sprinkle with sesame seeds and salt and pepper. To toast sesame seeds, place in an oven preheated to 350°F on a baking sheet and cook for about 5 minutes, or until the aroma is apparent.

Per serving: 52 Calories; 3g Fat (38% calories from fat); 3g Protein; 6g Carbohydrate; 0mg Cholesterol; 18mg Sodium

Spaghetti Squash Marinara

Serving Size: 6

1 medium spaghetti squash, about 3 1/2 lbs.
3 c. marinara sauce
1/3 c. grated Parmesan cheese
 salt and pepper to taste

Cut squash in half lengthwise and remove seeds. Place them cut side down in a large glass baking dish with a little water in it (about 1/2 cup). Cover dish with plastic wrap and microwave on high for 8 - 10 minutes or until squash is soft. Remove squash from pan and use a fork to remove the spaghetti like strands of squash. Heat marinara sauce. Place spaghetti squash on plates and top with sauce, then garnish with a sprinkling of Parmesan cheese.

Per serving: 114 Calories; 6g Fat (42% calories from fat); 4g Protein; 14g Carbohydrate; 4mg Cholesterol; 893mg Sodium

Spinach Pancakes

Serving Size: 5

3/8 c. skim milk
1 1/2 tsps. melted butter
1/4 c. all-purpose flour
1 eggs
1 tsp. maltitol
4 oz. frozen chopped spinach, squeezed dry
1 dash nutmeg
 salt and pepper to taste

Combine milk, butter, flour, egg, and malitol to make a batter. Add the spinach and seasonings. Heat a large nonstick skillet sprayed with nonstick cooking spray over medium heat. Place the desired amount of batter in the pan, and cook until both sides are golden brown, turning once. Serve immediately.

Notes: These pancakes are a great side dish - especially with a little Parmesan cheese sprinkled on top of them!

Per serving: 60 Calories; 2g Fat (32% calories from fat); 3g Protein; 8g Carbohydrate; 40mg Cholesterol; 49mg Sodium

Stir Fried Vegetables

Serving Size: 8

Nonstick cooking spray
1 clove garlic, crushed
1 tbsp. low sodium soy sauce
3 c. shredded cabbage
2 c. broccoli florets
1 c. sliced carrot
1 c. sliced green onions
2 c. fresh mushrooms, sliced
6 oz. snow peas, partially thawed
1 tbsp. cornstarch
2 tsps. chicken bouillon cubes or granules
1 c. water

Coat a wok or large skillet with nonstick cooking spray. Heat at medium heat or 300°F for 2 minutes. Add garlic and soy sauce. Stir fry 3 minutes. Add cabbage, broccoli, carrot and green onions. Stir fry 3-4 minutes or until vegetables are crisp-tender. Add mushrooms and snow peas. Stir fry 1 to 2 minutes more. In separate bowl, combine cornstarch, bouillon and water. Stir until dissolved. Pour over vegetables and continue to stir fry until thick and bubbly.

Per serving: 48 Calories; less than one gram Fat (7% calories from fat); 3g Protein; 9g Carbohydrate; 0mg Cholesterol; 440mg Sodium

Stuffed Artichokes

Serving Size: 8

4 fresh artichokes
1 1/2 c. seasoned bread crumbs
1/2 c. grated Parmesan cheese
1 tbsp. garlic powder
1 tsp. salt
2 tbsps. minced parsley
1/2 tsp. pepper
1/2 c. extra virgin olive oil

Preheat oven to 350°F. Wash artichokes and cut off all pointed tips on as many leaves as possible. Cut the stem from the bottom off so that the artichoke can stand up straight. Combine all other ingredients and place the stuffing between each of the leaves. Place the artichokes in a large baking pan and fill the pan with 1 inch of hot water. Place foil over the pan very tightly and bake for 1-1 1/2 hours or until the leaves open and are easily pulled off. Add more water to the pan if necessary.

Notes: The oil in this recipe can be reduced for a lower fat dish, but the stuffing will be a little drier.

Per serving: 265 Calories; 16g Fat (53% calories from fat); 8g Protein; 24g Carbohydrate; 5mg Cholesterol; 1042mg Sodium

Stuffed Bell Peppers

Serving Size: 4

4 medium bell peppers, red or green
1 tsp. canola oil
1/3 c. onion, chopped fine
2 c. fresh mushrooms, sliced
2 tsps. minced garlic
1 c. corn
2 eggs, beaten
1 c. low-fat ricotta cheese
4 tbsps. grated Parmesan cheese

Preheat oven to 350°F. Cut the tops off the bell peppers and remove the seeds and ribs from the inside. Set aside. Heat the oil in a large skillet over medium heat and add the onion and saute for five minutes or until they are soft, then add the mushrooms and garlic and saute until the mushrooms are soft, about 5 more minutes. Add corn to the skillet and saute for 3 minutes, stirring frequently. Add eggs, both cheeses and remove from heat while you combine everything. Place peppers in a baking dish and stuff with cheese mixture. Cover with foil and bake until bubbly, about 45 minutes.

Per serving: 202 Calories; 8g Fat (34% calories from fat); 15g Protein; 19g Carbohydrate; 122mg Cholesterol; 441mg Sodium

Summer Squash Noodles

Serving Size: 5

1 large yellow squash
1 large zucchini
1 leek
2 tsps. extra virgin olive oil
 salt and pepper to taste
1 tbsp. chopped fresh basil

Cut yellow squash and zucchini in half lengthwise and scoop out the seeds with a teaspoon. Lay the vegetables down as flat as possible and cut them into long strips, about 1/4" thin. Cut off the dark green part of the leek, and cut the remaining white part in half lengthwise. Under running water, wash in between the layers of the leek to get out all trapped dirt. Just like the squash, lay each half down flat, and slice into long strips, about 1/4" thick. Heat a 10 inch skillet, with the olive oil in it, over medium heat. Add the leeks, and stir frequently for about 3 minutes, or until the leeks soften up a little. Add the squash and zucchini and keep stirring, and cook about 5-8 minutes more, or until the vegetables are fork tender. Season the vegetables with salt and pepper, then remove from heat and stir in the basil. Serve hot.

Per serving: 31 Calories; 2g Fat (51% calories from fat); 1g Protein; 3g Carbohydrate; 0mg Cholesterol; 4mg Sodium

Sweet Glazed Carrots

Serving Size: 6

1 1/2 lbs. baby carrots
1 1/4 c. chicken stock
2 tbsps. brown sugar replacement
1 tbsp. butter
1/4 tsp. salt

Combine all ingredients in a 10 inch skillet over medium heat. Bring mixture to a simmer and cover. Simmer until carrots are almost done, about 7 minutes, then remove the lid. Increase heat to medium high and cook until liquids in pan are reduced to about 1/4 cup. If the carrots are cooked before the liquid is reduced this much, remove the carrots from the pan and finish reducing the liquid, then put them back in the pan to reheat them and coat them with the glaze.

Notes: Baby carrots are very handy in the kitchen because they eliminate the peeling and chopping process!

Per serving: 64 Calories; 3g Fat (35% calories from fat); 1g Protein; 10g Carbohydrate; 5mg Cholesterol; 595mg Sodium

Sweet Potato Casserole

Serving Size: 6

18 oz. canned sweet potatoes, drained
1 c. Sugar Twin brown sugar replacement, divided
1/4 c. skim milk
1 each egg
1 tbsp. reduced-calorie margarine, melted
1 tsp. vanilla
 Nonstick cooking spray
1 tbsp. flour
1 tbsp. reduced-calorie margarine

Combine sweet potatoes, 3/4 cup brown sugar replacement Twin, milk, egg, melted margarine and vanilla. Mix well. Spoon into shallow baking dish prepared with nonstick cooking spray. Combine flour with 1/4 cup brown sugar replacement Twin; cut in 1 tablespoon margarine until crumbly. Sprinkle over potatoes. Bake at 350°F for 35 minutes or until heated thoroughly.

Per serving: 102 Calories; 3g Fat (25% calories from fat); 2g Protein; 17g Carbohydrate; 30mg Cholesterol; 69mg Sodium

The Best (and Easiest) Green Beans You Will Ever Eat

Serving Size: 4

1 lb. green beans, must be fresh
1/4 tsp. salt
1/8 tsp. fresh ground black pepper
1 tbsp. butter

Cut ends off of green beans and cut into smaller pieces, if desired. Rinse beans. Bring a large pot of water to a full boil. Place the green beans in the water and let them boil for 8 minutes. Drain beans, and combine them with the salt, pepper and butter. Serve hot.

Per serving: 56 Calories; 3g Fat (42% calories from fat); 2g Protein; 7g Carbohydrate; 8mg Cholesterol; 168mg Sodium

Vegetable Casserole

Serving Size: 6

1 c. onions, diced
1 red pepper, diced
1 tbsp. salad oil
1 1/2 c. broccoli florets
4 carrots diced
8 oz. low sodium tomato juice
1 bay leaf
1/2 tsp. ground basil or 2 tsp fresh
 salt to taste
1 bunch spinach, chopped
2 tbsps. fresh parsley, chopped
2 c. mashed potatoes
 paprika

 Dice onion, dice pepper, peel and dice carrots, cut the broccoli into florets and stems. Wash spinach. Saute onion and peppers in oil in a large skillet. Add broccoli, carrots, tomato sauce, bay leaf, basil and salt to taste. Blend thoroughly. Bring to a boil, cover, reduce heat to simmer, and cook vegetables until just tender, about 15 minutes. Stir in spinach. Transfer to a 13 x 9 x 2-inch baking dish that has been sprayed with nonstick cooking spray. Blend parsley into prepared potatoes; spread over top of vegetables. Bake in preheated 350°F oven for 15 minutes. Serve hot.

Per serving: 132 Calories; 3g Fat (22% calories from fat); 4g Protein; 23g Carbohydrate; 1mg Cholesterol; 193mg Sodium

Vegetarian Moussaka

Serving Size: 6

1 large eggplant, sliced very thin
salt
1 tbsp. extra virgin olive oil
1 large onion, sliced very thin
2 cloves garlic, minced
2 large tomatoes, chopped
2 tsps. dried basil
2 tsps. dried oregano
1/2 c. vegetable broth
1 c. cooked chick peas
2 each eggs, beaten
1/4 c. grated Parmesan cheese

Preheat oven to 300°F. Place eggplant slices on a baking tray single layer and sprinkle with a little salt. Bake 10 - 15 minutes or until they are tender. Heat olive oil in a 10 inch skillet over medium heat and saute onion until soft, about 5 minutes. Ad garlic, herbs, tomatoes and vegetable broth. Saute about 10 minutes more, stirring frequently. Place eggplant in a 9X13 baking dish that has been sprayed with nonstick cooking spray. Turn oven temperature to 350°F. Spread chick peas over eggplant then top with beaten eggs. Place tomato mixture over eggs, then sprinkle with cheese. Bake for 45 minutes.

Per serving: 160 Calories; 6g Fat (34% calories from fat); 8g Protein; 20g Carbohydrate; 65mg Cholesterol; 243mg Sodium

Zucchini Casserole

Serving Size: 8

4 medium zucchini, sliced
3/4 c. shredded carrots
1/2 c. chopped onion
1/2 c. water
1/2 c. plain yogurt

Place zucchini in medium saucepan. Cover with water and cook for 5 minutes or until crisp-tender. Drain well and set aside. In large saucepan, combine carrot, onion and 1/2 cup water. Cover. Bring to boil. Reduce heat and simmer 10 minutes or until crisp-tender. Drain. Add yogurt and zucchini. Stir gently. Pour into 1 1/2 quart casserole dish that has been prepared with nonstick cooking spray. Bake at 350°F for 30 to 40 minutes or until done.

Per serving: 25 Calories; 1g Fat (19% calories from fat); 1g Protein; 4g Carbohydrate; 2mg Cholesterol; 12mg Sodium

Zucchini Casserole Special

Serving Size: 8

2 onion, thinly sliced
6 tbsps. reduced-calorie margarine
2 lbs. zucchini, thinly sliced
2 medium tomatoes, thinly sliced
Salt to taste
Pepper to taste
1/4 c. Parmesan cheese, grated

Saute onions in margarine until yellow. Add zucchini; cook for 5 minutes, stirring constantly. Add tomatoes, salt and pepper. Cover. Cook 5 additional minutes. Either reduce heat and cook until tender or transfer to casserole dish that has been prepared with nonstick cooking spray and sprinkle with cheese. Bake at 375°F for 45 to 60 minutes or until brown.

Per serving: 87 Calories; 5g Fat (50% calories from fat); 3g Protein; 9g Carbohydrate; 2mg Cholesterol; 158mg Sodium

Desserts

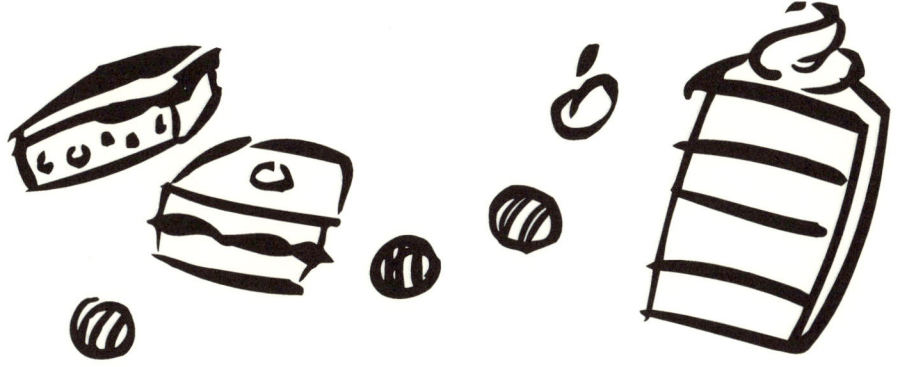

Apple Cinnamon Raisin Bread Pudding

Serving Size: 4

8 slices wheat bread
8 oz. egg substitute
1/4 c. brown sugar replacement
1/2 tsp. ground cinnamon
2 c. skim milk
1/2 tsp. vanilla
1/2 c. apples, finely chopped
1/3 c. golden raisins

Beat egg substitute, brown sugar replacement replacement, cinnamon, milk and vanilla in bowl. In 2 quart casserole dish that has been prepared with nonstick cooking spray, arrange in order: half the bread, 1/2 the apples, 1/2 the raisins and 1/2 the egg mixture; repeat layers in order. Set casserole dish in oven in large pan filled half way with boiling water. Bake at 350°F for 1 1/4 hours.

Per serving: 315 Calories; 9g Fat (25% calories from fat); 16g Protein; 45g Carbohydrate; 3mg Cholesterol; 443mg Sodium

Apple Crisp

Serving Size: 10

4 c. apples, peeled and sliced
1 tbsp. lemon juice
1/3 c. flour
1 c. quick-cooking oats
1/2 c. maltitol, honey flavored
1/2 tsp. salt
1 tsp. cinnamon
1/4 c. reduced-calorie margarine

Prepare a 9 inch pie pan with nonstick cooking spray. Layer apple slices evenly in pie pan. Sprinkle with lemon juice. In separate bowl combine remaining ingredients, mix well. Pour over apples slices. Bake at 375°F for 30 minutes or until golden brown.

Per serving: 118 Calories; 3g Fat (20% calories from fat); 2g Protein; 25g Carbohydrate; 0mg Cholesterol; 163mg Sodium

Apple Pudding

Serving Size: 6

3 medium apples, peeled and sliced
  Nonstick cooking spray
1 c. flour
1 tsp. baking powder
1/4 tsp. salt
1/3 c. reduced-calorie margarine
1/3 c. maltitol
1/2 tsp. lemon zest, grated
1/2 tsp. vanilla
1 egg
1/2 c. skim milk

Arrange apple slices in bottom of 8 inch square baking pan prepared with nonstick cooking spray. Set aside. In small bowl, combine flour, baking powder and salt. Set aside. In medium bowl, mix margarine, maltitol, lemon zest and vanilla. Beat at medium speed until well blended. Add egg; beat until fluffy. Alternately add flour and milk to margarine mixture, beginning and ending with flour. Pour over apples in prepared pan. Bake at 375°F for 40 to 45 minutes or until done. Cut into 6 squares and serve hot.

Per serving: 207 Calories; 6g Fat (25% calories from fat); 4g Protein; 38g Carbohydrate; 30mg Cholesterol; 293mg Sodium

Honey Cheese Crepes

Serving Size: 4

1/2 c. flour
2/3 c. skim milk
1 large egg white
1/2 c. nonfat cottage cheese
2 tsps. honey flavored maltitol
1/8 tsp. ginger
ground cinnamon to taste

Combine milk and egg white. Mix well. Add flour and stir to combine ingredients. Coat a nonstick skillet with nonstick cooking spray and set over moderately high heat. When hot, pour 2 tablespoons batter into pan, turning to make a thin pancake. Cook for 30 seconds on each side or until golden brown. Transfer to plate, layer with wax paper and repeat until batter is used up. Combine cottage cheese, honey, ginger and cinnamon until very smooth. Spread each crepe with 1 tablespoon of cheese mixture. Fold crepe in half and half again. Crepes can be made ahead of time and frozen. To freeze, stack between wax paper. Thaw before serving.

Per serving: 99 Calories; 0.2gram Fat (2.1% calories from fat); 7.6g Protein; 16.8g Carbohydrate; 2mg Cholesterol; 110mg Sodium

Maple-Glazed Apple Slices

Serving Size: 6

4 Golden Delicious apples
2 tbsps. reduced-calorie margarine
3 tbsps. maltitol-sweetened maple syrup
1 tbsp. water
1 tsp. fresh lemon juice
1/4 tsp. cinnamon

Peel and core apples. Cut into 1/4 inch thick slices. In medium skillet, heat butter over medium high heat until foam subsides. Add apples; saute until golden and tender, turning constantly. Stir in maple syrup, water, lemon juice, cinnamon and salt. Cook, stirring constantly, until apples are glazed.

Per serving: 64 Calories; 2g Fat (25% calories from fat); 0g Protein; 13g Carbohydrate; 0mg Cholesterol; 51mg Sodium

Old Fashioned Bread Pudding

Serving Size: 8

6 white bread slices, crusts removed
2 tbsps. reduced-calorie margarine, melted
3 tsps. Sugar Twin, divided
1 tsp. ground cinnamon
1/2 c. seedless raisins
Nonstick cooking spray
4 eggs beaten
2 c. skim milk
1 tsp. vanilla

Brush bread lightly with melted butter and sprinkle with 1 teaspoon Sugar Twin/cinnamon mixture. Quarter each bread slice. Alternately layer with raisins in 1 1/2 quart casserole dish that has been prepared with nonstick cooking spray. Set aside. Combine eggs, milk, vanilla, and remaining 2 teaspoons of Sugar Twin. Pour over bread. Place dish in pan containing 1 inch of hot water. Bake at 350°F for 55 to 60 minutes or until done. Serve warm or cover and refrigerate until chilled.

Per serving: 145 Calories; 4g Fat (27% calories from fat); 7g Protein; 20g Carbohydrate; 93mg Cholesterol; 195mg Sodium

Peanut Butter Fudge Crunchy Snack

Serving Size: 10

1/4 c. maltitol, honey flavored
2 tsps. maltitol-sweetened fudge sauce
1/4 c. peanut butter
2 1/2 c. Cheerios®
1/2 c. raisins
1/2 c. pretzels sticks

Combine maltitol and Fudge Sauce in small saucepan. Heat to boiling. Remove from heat and add peanut butter. In large bowl, combine cereal, raisins and pretzels. Pour chocolate mixture over cereal. Toss gently to coated evenly. Spread in 9x13 inch pan to cool.

Per serving: 143 Calories; 4g Fat (24% calories from fat); 4g Protein; 26g Carbohydrate; 0mg Cholesterol; 297mg Sodium

Angel Food Cake

Serving Size: 14

3/4 c. cake flour, sifted
12 oz. maltitol
1 c. egg whites, room temperature
1 teaspoon cream of tartar
1/4 tsp. salt
1 tsp. vanilla
1/2 tsp. almond extract

Beat egg whites until foamy. Add cream of tartar and salt. Continue to beat until soft, and moist peaks form when beater is lifted. Add Vanilla Nature Sweet about 2 tablespoons at a time, beating well after each addition. Add vanilla and almond extract. Add sifted flour slowly, approximately 1/4 cup at a time. Pour into 10 inch tube pan that has been prepared with nonstick cooking spray. Bake at 325°F for 1 hour or until done. Invert pan and let cool.

Per serving: 61 Calories; less than one gram Fat (1% calories from fat); 2g Protein; 15g Carbohydrate; 0mg Cholesterol; 66mg Sodium

Apple Cake

Serving Size: 16

1 1/4 c. whole wheat flour
1 1/4 c. flour
3/4 c. maltitol
2 tsps. baking soda
2 1/2 tsps. ground cinnamon
3/4 c. maltitol-sweetened maple syrup
4 egg whites
2 tsps. vanilla
4 c. Granny Smith apples, about 5 medium
1/2 c. raisins
1/2 c. chopped walnuts, optional

Combine dry ingredients and mix well. Add maple syrup, egg whites and vanilla. Fold in remaining ingredients. Coat 9x13 inch pan with nonstick cooking spray. Pour batter into pan, bake at 350°F for 30-35 minutes or until done. Cool cake at least 20 minutes. Cut into squares and serve warm or at room temperature.

Per serving: 170 Calories; 1g Fat (4% calories from fat); 4g Protein; 41g Carbohydrate; 0mg Cholesterol; 174mg Sodium

Banana Crunch Cake

Serving Size: 10

1 c. flour plus 2 tbsps.
1/2 c. whole wheat flour
1/2 c. maltitol
2 tsps. baking powder
1 c. mashed bananas, very ripe
1/4 c. reduced-calorie margarine, melted
2 egg whites
1 tsp. vanilla

Topping

3/4 c. quick-cooking oats
3 tbsps. brown sugar replacement
2 tbsps. chopped walnuts
2 tbsps. maltitol-sweetened maple syrup

Topping: Combine ingredients. Stir until moist and crumbly. Set aside.

Combine flours, brown sugar replacement Twin and baking powder. Mix well. Add bananas, margarine, egg whites and vanilla. Mix well. Spread batter in 9 inch round pan that has been prepared with nonstick cooking spray. Sprinkle topping over batter. Bake at 350°F for 30 minutes or until done. Cool cake for 10 minutes and drizzle with glaze.

Per serving: 163 Calories; 3g Fat (16% calories from fat); 4g Protein; 33g Carbohydrate; 0mg Cholesterol; 141mg Sodium

Black Forest Cake

Serving Size: 10

1 c. flour
1/2 c. rolled oats, ground to flour
3/4 c. maltitol
1/4 c. cocoa
1 tsp. baking soda
1 tsp. vanilla
1/4 c. maltitol-sweetened fudge sauce
1 1/2 tsps. white vinegar
1 c. water
20 oz. cherry pie filling, sugar free
 Cool Whip Lite®

Combine dry ingredients and mix well. In separate bowl, combine vanilla, chocolate syrup, vinegar and water. Add chocolate mixture to the dry ingredients and mix well.

Coat a 10 inch pan with nonstick cooking spray. Pour batter into pan and bake at 350°F for 15-20 minutes or until done. Cool cake to room temperature. Invert onto baking sheet. Fill the depression with the cherry pie filling. Pipe or spoon Cool Whip in ring around the outer edge of pie filling. Slice and serve immediately. Refrigerate remaining cake.

Per serving: 187 Calories; 1g Fat (4% calories from fat); 3g Protein; 50g Carbohydrate; 0mg Cholesterol; 136mg Sodium

Butterscotch Bundt Cake

Serving Size: 16

2 1/3 c. flour
2/3 c. oat bran
1 1/3 c. brown sugar replacement
1 tbsp. lecithin granules, plus 1 1/2 tsps.
1 1/4 tsps. baking soda
1 1/4 c. buttermilk
2 egg whites
2 tbsps. maltitol
2 tsps. vanilla

Combine flour, oat bran, brown sugar replacement Twin, lecithin and baking soda. Mix well. Press out any lumps with the back of spoon. In separate bowl, combine buttermilk, egg whites, maltitol and vanilla. Combine buttermilk and flour mixtures. Mix well. Spread batter in 12-cup bundt pan that has been prepared with nonstick cooking spray. Bake at 350°F for 40 minutes or until done. Cool in pan approximately 20 minutes. Then invert onto wire rack; cool completely. Transfer to serving plate. Glaze with maltitol-sweetened butterscotch sauce, if desired.

Per serving: 94 Calories; 1g Fat (8% calories from fat); 4g Protein; 20g Carbohydrate; 1mg Cholesterol; 126mg Sodium

Chocolate Raspberry Cake

Serving Size: 12

12 oz. maltitol-sweetened butterscotch sauce
1 c. cake flour sifted
1/2 c. unsweetened cocoa powder
1/4 tsp. salt
8 egg whites
1 tsp. cream of tartar
1/3 c. maltitol-sweetened raspberry sauce
1 c. maltitol-sweetened fudge sauce

Preheat oven to 350°F. Sift together flour, cocoa powder and salt. Set aside. Beat egg whites at medium speed until foamy. Add cream of tartar, Butterscotch Sauce and Raspberry Sauce. Sift 1/2 of flour mixture over egg whites. Fold in with spatula until just mixed. Repeat with remaining flour. Pour into two 9 inch cake pan that have been prepared with nonstick cooking spray and bottoms have been lined with wax paper. Bake at 350°F for 20 minutes or until done. Invert pans onto wire racks; cool. Place layer on serving plate. Top with thin layer of Fudge Sauce that has been heated in the microwave 20 seconds. Add second layer. Spread with Fudge Sauce.

Per serving: 168 Calories; 1.6g Fat (6.2% calories from fat); 3.8g Protein; 49.7g Carbohydrate; 0mg Cholesterol; 102mg Sodium

Low-fat Pound Cake

Serving Size: 16

5 tbsps. butter or margarine, reduced calorie
1/4 c. maltitol
3 egg whites
1 1/2 tsps. vanilla
1 2/3 c. flour
1/2 c. oat bran
1/2 tsp. baking soda
1 c. nonfat yogurt, lemon or vanilla flavor

Combine margarine and maltitol and beat until smooth. Add egg whites and vanilla, beat until smooth. In separate bowl, combine flour, oat bran and baking soda. Add flour mixture and yogurt to margarine mixture. Mix well.

Spread batter in 8x4 inch loaf pan that has been prepared with nonstick cooking spray. Bake at 350°F for 55 to 60 minutes or until done. Cool cake at room temperature for 20 minutes then invert pan onto wire rack to cool completely before serving.

Per serving: 107 Calories; 4g Fat (31% calories from fat); 3g Protein; 16g Carbohydrate; 10mg Cholesterol; 97mg Sodium

Maple Spice Cake

Serving Size: 16

1 1/3 c. flour
1 1/3 c. whole wheat flour
1 c. maltitol
1 tbsp. baking powder
1/2 tsp. ground ginger
1/4 tsp. ground nutmeg
1 1/3 c. skim milk
2/3 c. maltitol-sweetened maple syrup
4 egg whites

Mix flours, maltitol, baking powder and spices; add milk, maltitol-sweetened maple syrup and egg whites. Mix well. Coat 9x13 inch pan with nonstick cooking spray. Pour batter into pan and bake at 350°F for 30-35 minutes or until done. Cool to room temperature.
Frost with Fluffy Maple Frosting

Per serving: 152 Calories; less than one gram Fat (2% calories from fat); 4g Protein; 37g Carbohydrate; 0mg Cholesterol; 94mg Sodium

Mocha Fudge Cake

Serving Size: 16

2 c. flour
1 1/4 c. maltitol
1/2 c. cocoa
1 tsp. baking powder
1/2 tsp. baking soda
1/4 tsp. salt (optional)
3/4 c. unsweetened applesauce
1 2/3 c. coffee at room temperature
2 tsps. vanilla
1/2 c. chopped walnuts, optional

Combine dry ingredients, mixing well. In separate bowl, combine Prune butter, coffee and vanilla, mix well. Add prune mixture to flour mixture, mix well. Fold in walnuts. Spread batter in 9x13 inch pan that has been prepared with nonstick cooking spray. Bake at 350°F for 30 to 35 minutes or until done. Do not overbake. Cool to room temperature. Cut into squares to serve.

Per serving: 119 Calories; 1g Fat (7% calories from fat); 2g Protein; 30g Carbohydrate; 0mg Cholesterol; 97mg Sodium

Old Fashioned Strawberry Shortcake

Serving Size: 10

Biscuits

1 1/2 c. flour	1/2 c. oat bran
1/4 c. maltitol	1 tbsp. baking powder
4 tbsps. butter or margarine, low-fat	2/3 c. buttermilk
3 tbsps. egg substitute, liquid fat free	

Fruit Topping

3 c. fresh strawberries, sliced	1/3 c. maltitol

Cream Topping

1/2 c. nonfat vanilla yogurt	3/4 c. Cool Whip Lite®

Fruit Topping: Combine strawberries and maltitol. Cover and refrigerate several hours or overnight to allow juices to develop.

Cream Topping: Gently fold yogurt into whipped topping. Chill until ready to serve. Combine flour, oat bran, maltitol and baking powder. Mix well. Cut margarine into flour mixture with pastry cutter until dough resembles coarse crumbs. In separate bowl, combine egg substitute and buttermilk. Add to flour and stir until moistened. Drop heaping tablespoons of dough (enough to make 10 biscuits) onto cookie sheet that has been prepared with nonstick cooking spray. Place 3/4 inches apart for soft biscuits or 2 inches apart for crusty biscuits. To assemble shortcakes, slice each biscuit in half lengthwise and place on the bottom of individual serving plates or bowls. Top with 3 tablespoons of strawberries. Add top of biscuit and cover with 3 tablespoons of strawberries. Drop heaping tablespoon of cream topping on top and serve.

Per serving: 197 Calories; 7g Fat (26% calories from fat); 5g Protein; 38g Carbohydrate; 13mg Cholesterol; 193mg Sodium

Pear Crumble Cake

Serving Size: 8

2/3 c. flour
2/3 c. whole wheat flour
1/2 c. maltitol
1 1/2 tsps. baking powder
1/8 tsp. ground nutmeg
2/3 c. skim milk
1/4 c. prunes, pureed
1 egg white
1 1/2 c. fresh pears, peeled and sliced

Topping:
1/4 c. quick-cooking oats
2 tbsps. toasted wheat germ
2 tbsps. brown sugar replacement
1 tbsp. maltitol-sweetened maple syrup

To make topping, combine topping ingredients together until moist and crumbly. Set aside.

Combine dry ingredients. Mix well. Stir in milk, pureed prune and egg white. Pour batter into 9 inch round pan that has been prepared with nonstick cooking spray. Arrange pear slices in circular pattern over the batter. Sprinkle with topping. Bake at 350°F for 30 to 35 minutes or until done. Cool at least 20 minutes. To serve, cut into wedges and serve warm or at room temperature.

Per serving: 174 Calories; 1g Fat (4% calories from fat); 5g Protein; 42g Carbohydrate; 0mg Cholesterol; 87mg Sodium

Sweet Potato Snack Cake

Serving Size: 8

1 c. whole wheat flour
3/4 c. brown sugar replacement
2 tsps. baking powder
1/2 tsp. ground cinnamon
1/8 tsp. ground nutmeg
1 1/2 c. sweet potato, cooked and mashed
2 egg whites
2 tbsps. skim milk

Combine flour, brown sugar replacement Twin, baking powder and spices. Mix well. Add remaining ingredients. Mix well. Spread batter in 8 inch square pan that has been prepared with nonstick cooking spray. Bake at 325°F for 40 to 45 minutes or until done. Cool at room temperature.

Per serving: 76 Calories; less than one gram Fat (4% calories from fat); 3g Protein; 16g Carbohydrate; 0mg Cholesterol; 110mg Sodium

Brownies

Serving Size: 12

4 oz. unsweetened chocolate
1/3 c. reduced-calorie margarine
2 eggs
1 c. maltitol, plus 2 tbsps.
1/2 c. flour
1/2 c. nuts chopped
1 tsp. vanilla

Melt chocolate and butter together. Beat eggs with maltitol and add to chocolate. Add flour, blend, add nuts and vanilla. Stir until blended. Spread batter into 9 inch square pan that has been prepared with nonstick cooking spray. Bake at 350°F for 25 minutes or until done.

Notes: Can use maltitol-sweetened butterscotch sauce instead of maltitol for variety.

Per serving: 184 Calories; 12g Fat (49% calories from fat); 3g Protein; 24g Carbohydrate; 31mg Cholesterol; 73mg Sodium

Chocolate Oatmeal Jumbles

Serving Size: 42

1 c. whole wheat flour
1 c. quick-cooking oats
1/4 c. maltitol
2 tbsps. cocoa
1 tsp. baking soda
1/3 c. chocolate syrup, sugar free
1 tsp. vanilla
1/4 c. raisins
1/4 c. chopped walnuts
1/4 c. grain sweetened chocolate chips

Combine first 5 ingredients. Add chocolate syrup, water and vanilla and mix well. Stir in remaining ingredients. Spray cookie sheet with nonstick cooking spray. Drop rounded teaspoons of dough, approximately 1 1/2 teaspoons apart. Flatten slightly. Bake at 275°F for 18 to 20 minutes or until lightly brown. Cool on cookie sheets then transfer to wire racks. To store, keep in air tight container separating the layers with waxed paper.

Per serving: 34 Calories; 1g Fat (13% calories from fat); 1g Protein; 7g Carbohydrate; 0mg Cholesterol; 32mg Sodium

Chocolate Raspberry Treats

Serving Size: 42

4 tbsps. butter or margarine
3/4 c. brown sugar replacement
1/4 c. chocolate syrup, sugar free
1 tbsp. water plus 1 tsp.
1 tsp. vanilla
1 1/2 c. whole wheat flour
1 c. quick-cooking oats
2 tbsps. cocoa
3/4 tsp. baking soda
3 tbsps. raspberry jam, sugar free

In bowl of food processor or electric mixer, combine margarine and brown sugar replacement Twin. Process until smooth. Add chocolate syrup, water, and vanilla. Process until smooth. In separate bowl, combine flour, oats, cocoa and baking soda. Add flour to margarine mixture. Process until dough forms a ball and leaves the sides of the bowl. Roll dough into 1 inch balls. Place cookies 1 1/2 inch apart, on cookie sheet that has been prepared with nonstick cooking spray. Using the back of a 1/4 inch measuring spoon or your thumb, make a depression in the center of each cookie. Fill each depression with 1/4 tsp. jam. Bake at 300°F for 18 to 20 minutes or until bottoms are golden. Cool for 1 minute and then transfer to wire racks to cool completely. Serve immediately or store in air tight container, separating the layers with wax paper.

Per serving: 40 Calories; 1g Fat (29% calories from fat); 1g Protein; 7g Carbohydrate; 3mg Cholesterol; 35mg Sodium

Colossal Chocolate Chippers

Serving Size: 30

3/4 c. whole wheat flour
1/2 c. flour
2/3 c. brown sugar replacement
3/4 tsp. baking soda
1/4 c. prunes, pureed
2 tbsps. maltitol
1 tsp. vanilla
1/3 c. grain sweetened chocolate chips
1/3 c. chopped walnuts, optional

Combine flours, Sugar Twin and baking soda; mix well. Add prune puree, maltitol and vanilla. Mix well. Stir in chocolate chips and nuts if desired. Drop slightly rounded teaspoons onto cookie sheet that has been prepared with nonstick cooking spray. Bake 350°F for 9 minutes or until golden. Cool for about 1 minutes on pan then transfer to wire racks to cool completely. Serve immediately or store in air tight container with layers separated by wax paper.

Notes: Chocolate chips sweetened with grain sweeteners such as malted barley can be found at most health food stores.

Per serving: 33 Calories; 1g Fat (18% calories from fat); 1g Protein; 6g Carbohydrate; 0mg Cholesterol; 32mg Sodium

Cranberry Spice Cookies

Serving Size: 42

1 c. whole wheat flour
3/4 c. flour plus 2 tbsps.
2/3 c. maltitol
1 tsp. baking soda
1/2 tsp. ground cinnamon
1/8 tsp. ground nutmeg
1/3 c. prunes, pureed
1/4 c. maltitol
1 tsp. vanilla
1/2 c. cranberries, dried
1 c. oat flakes

Combine flours, maltitol, baking soda and spices. Mix well. Add pureed prunes, maltitol and vanilla. Mix well. Stir in cranberries or raisins and cereal flakes. Drop rounded teaspoons on cookie sheet prepared with nonstick cooking spray. Flatten slightly. Bake at 350°F for 9 minutes or until golden. Cool on pan 1 minute, then remove to wire racks to cool completely. Serve immediately or store in air tight container, separating layers with wax paper.
Notes: Raisins can be substituted for dried cranberries, if you wish.

Per serving: 38 Calories; less than one gram Fat (2% calories from fat); 1g Protein; 10g Carbohydrate; 0mg Cholesterol; 40mg Sodium

Fudge Frosted Oatmeal Cookies

Serving Size: 60

1 c. margarine
1/3 c. brown sugar replacement
1/2 c. maltitol, honey flavored
1 egg
2 tsps. vanilla
1 1/2 c. flour
1 tsp. baking soda
1/2 tsp. salt
1 tsp. cinnamon
3 c. quick-cooking oats
2 tbsps. apple juice

Beat margarine, Sugar Twin and maltitol until light and fluffy. Add egg, vanilla and juice. In separate bowl, combine flour, baking soda, salt and cinnamon. Mix in dry ingredients. Beat on low until moist. Stir oats. Drop by rounded teaspoons onto cookie sheet prepared with nonstick cooking spray. Bake at 375°F for 15 minutes or until done. While cookies are cooling, heat 1/2 c. maltitol-sweetened fudge sauce. Drizzle 1/4 tsp. over each cookie.

Per serving: 60 Calories; 3g Fat (49% calories from fat); 1g Protein; 7g Carbohydrate; 3mg Cholesterol; 75mg Sodium

Fudgy Cocoa Brownies

Serving Size: 16

1/2 c. prunes, pureed
3/4 c. maltitol
3 egg whites
1/4 c. cocoa plus 2 tbsps.
1/4 c. flour plus 2 tbsps.
1/4 c. oat bran
1/8 tsp. salt, optional
1 tsp. vanilla
1/3 c. chopped pecans, optional

Combine prune puree, maltitol and egg whites; mix well. Add remaining ingredients and stir well. Spread batter in 8 inch square pan that has been prepared with nonstick cooking spray. Bake at 375°F for 23 to 25 minutes or until done. Cool to room temperature, cut into squares and serve.

Notes: For the pureed prunes, you can purchase them already pureed in health food sections or as baby food.

Prune butter is harder to find, but can be used just like prune puree.

Per serving: 62 Calories; 1g Fat (13% calories from fat); 2g Protein; 15g Carbohydrate; 0mg Cholesterol; 27mg Sodium

Georgia's Fudge Bars

Serving Size: 16

1/3 c. flour
1/3 c. oat bran
1/3 c. cocoa
1 c. maltitol
1/8 tsp. salt, optional
1/2 c. sweet potatoes, cooked and mashed
3 egg whites
1 tsp. vanilla
1/3 c. chopped pecans, optional

Combine flour, oat bran, cocoa, maltitol, and salt if desired. Mix well. Add sweet potatoes, egg whites and vanilla. Mix well. Fold in nuts. Spread in 8 inch square pan that has been prepared with nonstick cooking spray. Bake at 325°F for 25 minutes or until done. Cool to room temperature, cut and serve.

Per serving: 67 Calories; 1g Fat (13% calories from fat); 2g Protein; 17g Carbohydrate; 0mg Cholesterol; 28mg Sodium

Great Pumpkin Cookies

Serving Size: 38

1 c. whole wheat flour
1 c. oat bran
3/4 c. brown sugar replacement
3/4 tsp. baking soda
1/2 c. pumpkin, cooked and mashed
1/4 c. maltitol-sweetened maple syrup

Coating
2 tbsps. pecans, finely ground
2 tbsps. maltitol

Coating: Combine pecans with maltitol in small bowl. Mix well and set aside.

Combine flour, oat bran, brown sugar replacement Twin and baking soda. Mix well. Add pumpkin and maple syrup. Roll dough into 1 inch balls and roll in pecan mixture until coated. Place 1 1/2 inch apart on cookie sheet prepared with nonstick cooking spray. Flatten each cookie to 1/4 inch with bottom of glass. Bake at 300°F for 15 minutes or until golden. Cool 1 minute and then transfer to wire rack to cool completely. Serve immediately or store in air tight container, separating layers with wax paper.

Per serving: 23 Calories; less than one gram Fat (11% calories from fat); 1g Protein; 6g Carbohydrate; 0mg Cholesterol; 25mg Sodium

Light and Luscious Brownies

Serving Size: 16

6 tbsps. margarine
1 c. maltitol
3 egg whites
1 tsp. vanilla
3/4 c. flour
1/3 c. cocoa
1/3 c. chopped nuts, optional

Melt margarine in medium sized sauce pan over low heat. Remove from heat and add maltitol. Then add egg whites and vanilla. Stir in flour and cocoa. Fold in nuts. Spread batter in 8 inch square pan that has been prepared with nonstick cooking spray. Bake at 325°F for 25 minutes or until done. Cool to room temperature.

Per serving: 120 Calories; 6g Fat (41% calories from fat); 2g Protein; 18g Carbohydrate; 0mg Cholesterol; 61mg Sodium

Oatmeal Raisin Cookies

Serving Size: 40

1 c. whole wheat flour
1 1/2 c. quick-cooking oats
1/2 c. brown sugar replacement
1 tsp. baking soda
1/4 c. prunes, pureed
1/4 c. maltitol plus 2 tbsps.
1 tsp. vanilla
1/2 c. raisins
1/2 c. chopped walnuts, optional

Combine flour, oats, Sugar Twin and baking soda; mix well. Add prune puree, maltitol and vanilla. Mix well. If dough is crumbly, keep mixing until it holds its shape. Stir in raisins and nuts if desired. Bake at 350°F for 9 minutes or until golden. Cool on pan for about 1 minute and then remove to wire racks and cool completely. Serve immediately or store in air tight container, separating layers with wax paper.

Per serving: 35 Calories; less than one gram Fat (11% calories from fat); 1g Protein; 7g Carbohydrate; 0mg Cholesterol; 32mg Sodium

Sugar-Free Oatmeal Cookies

Serving Size: 48

1 c. whole wheat flour
1 c. quick-cooking oats
1 tsp. ground cinnamon
1 tsp. baking powder
1/2 tsp. baking soda
1/4 tsp. ground nutmeg
1/4 tsp. ground allspice
1/4 tsp. ground cloves
1/2 c. raisins
1 c. unsweetened applesauce
1/4 c. water
1/3 c. vegetable oil
2 eggs
1 tsp. vanilla
1/4 c. nuts finely chopped

Combine all ingredients. Mix well. Drop by spoonfuls onto cookie sheet that has been prepared with nonstick cooking spray. Bake at 375°F for 10 to 15 minutes or until browned.

Per serving: 43 Calories; 2g Fat (46% calories from fat); 1g Protein; 5g Carbohydrate; 8mg Cholesterol; 24mg Sodium

Sweetie Bars

Serving Size: 2

3 graham crackers
1 tbsp. maltitol-sweetened fudge sauce
2 tbsps. peanut butter

Mix peanut butter and fudge sauce together. Spread on graham crackers.

Per serving: 157 Calories; 9.5g Fat (48.9% calories from fat); 4.7g Protein; 17.7g Carbohydrate; 0mg Cholesterol; 144mg Sodium

The Best Cake Brownies

Serving Size: 36

4 squares unsweetened baking chocolate (1 oz. each)
1 1/2 c. maltitol
1/2 c. egg substitute plus 1 tbsp.
1/2 c. buttermilk
3/4 c. prunes, pureed
2 tsps. vanilla
1 1/2 c. flour
1/4 tsp. salt, optional
3/4 c. chopped walnuts, optional

To melt chocolate in microwave: Place chocolate in microwaveable mixing bowl and microwave, uncovered on high, 3 to 4 minutes or until almost melted. Remove from oven and stir until completely melted.
Stove: Place chocolate in small saucepan and cook over low heat, stirring constantly until melted.
To melted chocolate, add maltitol, egg substitute, milk, pureed prunes and vanilla. Mix well. Add flour and if desired, salt and nuts. Pour batter into 9x13 inch pan prepared with nonstick cooking spray. Bake at 325°F for 35 to 40 minutes or until done. Cool to room temperature, cut into squares and serve.

Per serving: 77 Calories; 3g Fat (26% calories from fat); 2g Protein; 15g Carbohydrate; 0mg Cholesterol; 26mg Sodium

Thumbprint Cookies

Serving Size: 36

4 tbsps. margarine

1/2 c. maltitol, plus 2 tbsps.

3 tbsps. frozen orange juice concentrate, thawed

1 tsp. vanilla or almond extract

1 c. flour, plus 2 tbsps.

3/4 c. oat bran

3/4 c. baking soda

1/3 c. nuts, finely ground

3 tbsps. jam, sugar free

In bowl of food processor or electric mixer, combine margarine and maltitol. Process until smooth. Add the juice concentrate and vanilla. Process until smooth. In separate bowl, combine flour, oat bran and baking soda. Combine flour and margarine mixture. Process until dough forms a ball and leaves the sides of the bowl. Roll dough into 1 inch balls and roll in ground nuts. Place cookies 1 1/2 inch apart, on cookie sheet that has been prepared with nonstick cooking spray. Using the back of a 1/4 inch measuring spoon or your thumb, make a depression in the center of each cookie. Fill each depression with 1/4 teaspoon fruit spread. Bake at 300°F for 18 to 20 minutes or until bottoms are golden. Cool for 1 minute and then transfer to wire racks to cool completely. Serve immediately or store in air tight container, separating the layers with wax paper.

Per serving: 51 Calories; 2g Fat (34% calories from fat); 1g Protein; 9g Carbohydrate; 0mg Cholesterol; 1274mg Sodium

Ultimate Oatmeal Cookies

Serving Size: 42

6 tbsps. butter or margarine, low calorie
1/4 c. brown sugar replacement
1/2 c. maltitol
3 tbsps. egg substitute
1 tsp. vanilla
1 c. whole wheat flour
1 c. quick-cooking oats
1/2 tsp. baking soda
1/2 c. raisins
1/4 c. nuts chopped, optional

In bowl of food processor or electric mixer, combine margarine, brown sugar replacement, maltitol, egg substitute, and vanilla. Process until smooth. In separate bowl, combine flour and baking soda. Add flour to margarine mixture, mix well. Stir in remaining ingredients.

Drop by rounded teaspoons, 1 1/2 inch apart, on cookie sheet that has been prepared with nonstick cooking spray. Bake at 300°F for 15 to 18 minutes or until golden. Cool for 1 minute and then transfer to wire racks to cool completely. Serve immediately or store in air tight container, separating the layers with wax paper.

Notes: Instead of using raisins, try chopped dried apples, apricots, or dried cranberries or blueberries for a new twist!

Per serving: 50 Calories; 2g Fat (39% calories from fat); 1g Protein; 7g Carbohydrate; 4mg Cholesterol; 34mg Sodium

Whole Wheat Chocolate Chippers

Serving Size: 40

6 tbsps. margarine

1/4 c. brown sugar replacement

1/2 c. maltitol

3 tbsps. egg substitute

1 tsp. vanilla

1 1/4 c. whole wheat flour

1/2 tsp. baking soda

1/2 c. grain sweetened chocolate chips

1/3 c. walnuts, chopped

Process margarine, brown sugar replacement Twin, maltitol, egg substitute and vanilla in bowl of a food processor or blender until smooth. In separate bowl, combine flour and baking soda. Add flour to margarine mixture, process to mix well. Stir in remaining ingredients. Drop by rounded teaspoons 1 1/2 inches apart onto cookie sheet that has been prepared with nonstick cooking spray. Bake at 300°F for 16 minutes or until golden. Cool for 1 minute and transfer to wire racks to cool completely. Serve immediately or store in air tight container, separating layers with wax paper.

Per serving: 47 Calories; 3g Fat (44% calories from fat); 1g Protein; 6g Carbohydrate; 0mg Cholesterol; 38mg Sodium

Fluffy Maple Frosting

Serving Size: 16

1 c. maltitol-sweetened maple syrup
2 egg whites

Boil maple syrup in small saucepan over medium heat without stirring until temperature reaches 240°F or soft ball on candy thermometer. While heating syrup, beat the egg whites to soft peak. Slowly add the syrup to egg whites while beating on high speed. Beat for 5 minutes or until the icing is glossy and firm. Spread on cooled cake and serve immediately or refrigerate to prevent frosting from separating.

Per serving: 32 Calories; 0g Fat (0% calories from fat); 0g Protein; 10g Carbohydrate; 0mg Cholesterol; 10mg Sodium

Luscious Lemon Sauce

Serving Size: 4

1 c. maltitol
1 1/4 tbsps. cornstarch
pinch salt
1 1/4 c. cold water
3 1/2 tbsps. reduced-calorie margarine
4 tbsps. fresh lemon juice
3 tbsps. lemon zest, grated

Combine cornstarch and water in double boiler. Add salt and maltitol, cook, whisking gently, 2 to 3 minutes or until thickened. Add margarine, lemon juice and rind. Continue to cook 5 minutes, stirring constantly. Cool before serving.

Per serving: 193 Calories; 5g Fat (17% calories from fat); 0g Protein; 52g Carbohydrate; 0mg Cholesterol; 125mg Sodium

Apple Pie

Serving Size: 8

3 Granny Smith apples
1 c. maltitol
2 tbsps. reduced-calorie margarine
2 tbsps. cornstarch
2 tbsps. raisins, optional
　Nutmeg to taste
　Cinnamon to taste

Peel, core and slice apples. Mix with remaining ingredients and pour into prepared 9 inch pie shell. Bake on cooking sheet at 400°F for 45 minutes or until done.

Per serving: 118 Calories; 1g Fat (9% calories from fat); 0g Protein; 34g Carbohydrate; 0mg Cholesterol; 36mg Sodium

Banana Cream Pie

Serving Size: 8

1/2 c. maltitol
3 tbsps. cornstarch
1 pinch ground nutmeg
2 c. skim milk
1/4 c. egg substitute plus 2 tbsps.
1 tsp. vanilla
1 pie crust
3 large banana, sliced 1/4-inch thick
  Ground nutmeg, optional

Combine maltitol, cornstarch and nutmeg in medium saucepan. Slowly add milk. Place over medium heat and cook, stirring constantly with wire whisk until mixture comes to a boil. Reduce heat to low and cook another minute or 2 while stirring constantly. Blend 1/2 cup of the hot mixture with the egg substitute. Return mixture to saucepan. Cook, stirring constantly, over low heat for 2 to 3 minutes more. Do not allow the mixture to boil. Remove from heat, add vanilla. Let cool 15 minutes, stirring every 5 minutes. Spread a thin layer of filling over the bottom of the prepared pie crust. Top with half of the bananas and half the filling. Repeat, ending with filling. Sprinkle the top lightly with nutmeg, if desired.
Chill several hours or until set. Cut into wedges, and serve cold.

Per serving: 206 Calories; 7g Fat (29% calories from fat); 5g Protein; 35g Carbohydrate; 1mg Cholesterol; 193mg Sodium

Crunchy Cereal Pie Crust

Serving Size: 8

5 oz. oat flakes or oat flakes with almonds, about 2 1/2 c. ready to eat cereal

3 tbsps. jam, sugar free

In a food processor or blender, process cereal to fine crumbs. Measure the crumbs to make sure that there are about 1 1/4 cups of crumbs. Return the crumbs to the processor and add the fruit spread. Continue to process until moist and crumbly. Coat a 9 inch pie pan with nonstick cooking spray. Using the back of a spoon, press the crumbs against the sides and bottom of the pan forming an even crust. Bake shell at 350°F for 10-12 minutes or until edges are firm and dry. Cool to room temperature. Fill as desired.

Per serving: 95 Calories; less than one gram Fat (0.3% calories from fat); 2.4g Protein; 11g Carbohydrate; 0mg Cholesterol; 3mg Sodium

Key Lime Pie

Serving Size: 8

1 c. maltitol
1/4 c. flour
3 tbsps. cornstarch
2 c. water
3 large eggs, separated
1 tbsp. reduced-calorie margarine
1/4 c. fresh lime juice
lime zest from one lime
1 9 inch pie crust, baked

Beat egg yolks until creamy. Set aside. Combine maltitol, flour and cornstarch in saucepan. Gradually add water, stirring constantly. Cook, stirring constantly, until thickened. Gradually add egg yolks to mixture. Continue to stir constantly and return to low heat and cook 2 minutes. Add margarine, lime juice and zest. Cool. Pour into pie shell.

Notes: To get the zest from citrus fruits, grate only the colored part of the rind being careful not to include any of the bitter white pith.

Per serving: 226 Calories; 8g Fat (30% calories from fat); 4g Protein; 41g Carbohydrate; 69mg Cholesterol; 185mg Sodium

Lemon Chess Pie

Serving Size: 8

3/4 c. maltitol
1/2 c. cornstarch
1 3/4 c. buttermilk
1 tbsp. lemon zest
1/2 c. egg substitute
1/3 c. fresh lemon juice
1 pie crust

Combine maltitol and cornstarch in medium sized saucepan. Slowly add buttermilk, stirring constantly. Over medium heat, cook until thickened and bubbly with wire whisk. Add lemon rind and continue to cook for another 2 minutes. Reduce heat and blend about 1/2 cup of the hot mixture into the egg substitute. Return egg mixture to saucepan. Cook 2 to 3 minutes more, stirring constantly. Do not allow mixture to boil. Remove from heat and stir in lemon juice. Pour into pie crust.

Chill for several hours or until set. Cut into wedges and serve cold.

Per serving: 230 Calories; 8g Fat (29% calories from fat); 5g Protein; 39g Carbohydrate; 2mg Cholesterol; 233mg Sodium

Meringue

Serving Size: 8

3 egg whites
1/4 tsp. cream of tartar
6 tbsps. maltitol

Beat egg whites until light and frothy. Add cream of tartar and beat until stiff. Gradually add maltitol and beat until glossy. Layer meringue onto cooled pie, spreading to reach the edges. Bake at 425°F for 5 to 6 minutes or until tips turn golden brown.
Notes: Great on Key Lime Pie.

Per serving: 32 Calories; 0g Fat (0% calories from fat); 1g Protein; 9g Carbohydrate; 0mg Cholesterol; 21mg Sodium

Pecan Pie

Serving Size: 8

1 1/2 c. maltitol
1/4 c. reduced-calorie margarine
1 large egg
2 large egg whites
1 tbsp. vanilla
1 tsp. instant coffee
1/2 c. pecans
1 9 inch pie crust

Warm the maltitol and margarine together, enough to melt margarine. Add remaining ingredients except pecans. Mix well. Pour into pie shell. Top with pecans. Bake at 375°F for 45 minutes or until done.

Per serving: 268 Calories; 12g Fat (34% calories from fat); 3g Protein; 47g Carbohydrate; 23mg Cholesterol; 236mg Sodium

Pumpkin Pie

Serving Size: 8

2 c. canned pumpkin
3/4 c. maltitol
1 1/2 c. low-fat evaporated milk
2 large eggs
1 1/2 tsps. cinnamon
1/4 tsp. ground cloves
1 tsp. ginger
1 9 inch pie crust

Combine all ingredients. Pour into pie crust. Bake on lower shelf for 10 minutes at 450°F, lower temperature to 400°F and continue to cook 30 minutes or until done.

Per serving: 227 Calories; 7g Fat (27% calories from fat); 7g Protein; 39g Carbohydrate; 48mg Cholesterol; 218mg Sodium

Sugar Free Pecan Pudding Pie

Serving Size: 8

3 oz. instant vanilla pudding mix, sugar free
3/4 c. maltitol, honey flavored
3/4 c. low-fat evaporated milk
1 egg, slightly beaten
1 c. pecans, chopped or halves
1 8-inch pastry shell, uncooked

Blend pudding mix with maltitol. Gradually add milk and egg. Stir to blend. Pour into pie shell and top with pecans. Bake at 375°F for 40 minutes or until top is firm and begins to crack. Cool.

Per serving: 259 Calories; 11g Fat (35% calories from fat); 4g Protein; 41g Carbohydrate; 23mg Cholesterol; 251mg Sodium

Appendix

Sugar Terms:

Brown sugar	a soft sugar in which crystals are covered by a refined dark syrup
Carbohydrate	a nutrient made up of sugars and starches
Corn Sugar	a sugar made by the breakdown of cornstarch
Corn Syrup	a containing several types of sugars resulting from the breakdown of cornstarch
Dextrin	a sugar formed by the partial breakdown of starch
Dextrose	another name for sugar
Fructose	a simple sugar found in honey, fruit and juices
Galactose	a simple sugar found in milk sugar or lactose
Glucose	a simple sugar found in blood created by food, and used by the body for heat and energy
Honey	a sweet substance created naturally by bees
Invert Sugar	a sugar combination found in fruit
Lactose	a sugar found in milk
Levulose	another name for fruit sugar
Maltitol	a natural derivative of corn
Maltose	a crystalline sugar formed by the breakdown of starch
Mannitol	a sugar alcohol
Mannose	a sugar derived from manna and the ivory nut
Maple Sugar	a sugar from concentrated sugar maple sap
Molasses	a thick syrup created from raw sugar in the manufacturing of sugar
Sorbitol	a sugar alcohol
Sorghum	a syrup from sorghum grain
Starch	a complex chain of sugars usually found the a powdery form
Sucrose	another name for table sugar
Sugar	a carbohydrate, group includes the monosaccharides: fructose, galactose, glucose; and the disaccharides: sucrose, maltose and lactose
Xylose	a wood sugar from in corn cobs, straw, bran woodgum, seed bran, cherries, pears, peaches and plums
Xylitol	a sugar alcohol

Fat List:

Each serving on this list, contains about 5 grams of fat and 45 calories. In your daily intake, you can modify your fat intake by eating unsaturated fats instead of saturated ones.

Avocado	1/8 medium
Margarine	1 teaspoon
Margarine, diet**	1 tablespoon
Mayonnaise	1 teaspoon
Mayonnaise, reduced-calorie**	1 tablespoon
Nuts and seeds:	
Almonds, dry roasted	6 whole
Cashews, dry roasted	1 tablespoon
Peanuts	20 small or 10 large
Pecans	2 whole
Walnuts	2 whole
Other nuts	1 tablespoon
Seeds, pine nuts, sunflower (without shells)	1 tablespoon
Pumpkin seeds	2 teaspoons
Oil (corn, cottonseed, safflower, soybean sunflower, olive, peanut)	1 teaspoon
Olives**	10 small or 5 large
Salad dressing, mayonnaise-type	2 teaspoons
Salad dressing, mayonnaise-type, reduced-calorie	1 tablespoon
Salad dressing (oil varieties)**	1 tablespoon
Salad dressing, reduced-calorie	2 tablespoons

Saturated Fats:

Butter	1 teaspoon
Bacon**	1 slice
Chitterlings	1/2 ounce
Coconut, shredded	2 tablespoons
Coffee whitener, liquid	2 tablespoons
Coffee whitener, powder	4 teaspoons
Cream (light, coffee, table)	2 tablespoons
Cream, sour	2 tablespoons
Cream (heavy, whipping)	1 tablespoon
Cream cheese	1 tablespoon
Salt pork**	1/4 ounce

one serving contains 400 milligrams or more of sodium

two or more servings provides 400 milligrams or more of sodium

Selected Vendors and Suppliers:

Steels's Gourmet Foods
Continental Business Center
Suite D-175
Bridgeport, PA 19405
1-800-6-STEELS
Supplier of maltitol and maltitol-sweetened products

Leroux Creek
970 3100 Road
Hotchkiss, CO 81419
(970) 872-2256
Supplier of unsweetened applesauce and quality food products

Truffle Hound Gourmet, Inc.
1324 Pin Oak Rd.
Katy, TX 77494
(281) 395-2073
Supplier of plain and flavored pastas

Penzeys, Ltd.
1921 S. West Avenue
Waukesha, WI 53186
(414) 574-0277
Supplier of spices, seasonings and vanilla

Fredericksburg Herb Farm
P.O. Drawer 927
Fredericksburg, TX 78624
(21) 997-8615
Supplier of fresh and dried herbs; herb mixes

Chile Today - Hot Tamale
2-D Great Meadow Lane
East Hanover, NJ 07936
1-800-HOT-PEPPER
Supplier of chili products

Index

A

Angel Food Cake 248
Appetizers
    Artichoke Dip 7
    Artichoke Dip 2 8
    Artichoke Heart Spread 10
    Artichoke Pita Chips 10
    Baked Fried Zucchini and Mushrooms .. 11
    Billie Jo's Chicken Wings 12
    Black Bean Dip 13
    Black Bean Dip 2 14
    Caponata 15
    Cheese and Artichoke Dip 16
    Cold Veggie Platter 17
    Corned Beef and Cheese Dip 18
    Crab Appetizer 18
    Crab Devils 19
    Crab Spread 20
    Crabmeat Dip 21
    Creamy Salsa 22
    Curry Dip 22
    Dill Dip 23
    Guacamole 24
    Honey Mustard Dip 25
    Hot and Spicy Tomato Salsa 26
    Hot Bean Dip 27
    Hot Crab Dip 28
    Mexican Layer Dip 29
    Mushrooms Florentine 30
    Nacho Cheese Dip 31
    Onion Cheese Puffs 32
    Onion Spread 32
    Oven Zucchini Fries 33
    Pepper Cheese Dip 34
    Salmon Tortilla Appetizers 35
    Spinach and Cheese Bites 36
    Spinach Dip 37
    Spinach Dip 2 38
    Stuffed Mushrooms 39
    Tamale Balls 40
    The Best 7 layer Mexican Dip 41
    Tomato-Mozzarella Bites 42
    Tomatoes Stuffed with Salmon 43
    Tortilla Roll-Ups 44
    Vegetable Dip with Zip 45
    Vegetable Quesadillas 46
Apple Cake 249
Apple Cinnamon Raisin Bread Pudding . 241
Apple Crisp 242
Apple Pie 279
Apple Pudding 243
Apricot-Baked Chicken 173
Artichoke Dip 7
Artichoke Dip 2 8
Artichoke Heart Spread 9
Artichoke Pita Chips 10
Asparagus Torta 197

B

Baked Acorn Squash 198
Baked Fish With Vegetables 150
Baked Fried Zucchini and Mushrooms 11
Baked Halibut 151
Baked Pasta Primavera 113
Balsamic Marinated Vegetables 199
Banana Cream Pie 280
Banana Crunch Cake 250
Bean and Cabbage Soup 63
Bean and Pasta Stew 64
Beef and Cornbread Casserole 141
Beef in Mushroom Sauce 142
Billie Jo's Chicken Wings 12
Black Bean and Pork Stew 167
Black Bean Chili 65
Black Bean Dip 13
Black Bean Dip 2 14
Black Forest Cake 251
Blue Cheese Dressing 105
Boiled Parslied New Potatoes 200
Breads
    Buttermilk Whole Wheat Bread 49

Fat-Free French Bread 50
Focaccia 51
Garlic Bread 53
Nutty Wheat Bread 54
Peach Perfect Muffins 55
Pita Pizzas 56
Pretzels 57
Strawberry Oatmeal Muffins 58
Sugar Free Sticky Buns 59
Vegetable Pizza Crust 60
Broccoli with Pearl Onions Casserole 201
Broiled Sole with Cheese 152
Broiled Swordfish with Mango Salsa 153
Broiled Tomatoes with Horseradish 202
Brown Rice with Vegetables 114
Brownies 260
Buttermilk Herb Dressing 106
Buttermilk Mashed Potatoes 203
Buttermilk Whole Wheat Bread 49
Butterscotch Bundt Cake 252

C

Cabbage Casserole 204
Caponata 15
Cheddar Pea Salad 87
Cheese and Artichoke Dip 16
Chicken and Apples Over Fettucini 174
Chicken and Avocado Sandwich 129
Chicken Cacciatore 175
Chicken Corn Chowder 66
Chicken Dijon 176
Chicken Divan 177
Chicken Fajitas 178
Chicken Garlic Sticks 179
Chicken Pomodoro 180
Chicken Roasted with
    Rosemary and Garlic 181
Chicken Salad 88
Chicken with Pesto 182
Chicken-flavored Vegetable Soup 67

Chili Topped Potatoes 205
Chocolate Oatmeal Jumbles 261
Chocolate Raspberry Cake 253
Chocolate Raspberry Treats 262
Cold Veggie Platter 17
Colossal Chocolate Chippers 263
Corn and Bean Salad 89
Corn Relish 98
Corned Beef and Cheese Dip 18
Crab Appetizer 18
Crab Devils 19
Crab or Shrimp Salad 90
Crab Spread 20
Crabmeat Dip 21
Cranberry Spice Cookies 264
Cream of Onion Soup 68
Cream of Vegetable Soup 69
Creamy Green Beans 206
Creamy Linguini 115
Creamy Salsa 22
Crunchy Cereal Pie Crust 281
Curried Chicken 183
Curry Dip 22

D

Desserts
    Apple Cinnamon Raisin
        Bread Pudding 241
    Apple Crisp 242
    Apple Pudding 243
    Caakes
        Maple Spice Cake 255
    Cakes
        Angel Food Cake 248
        Apple Cake 249
        Banana Crunch Cake 250
        Black Forest Cake 251
        Butterscotch Bundt Cake 252
        Chocolate Raspberry Cake 253
        Low-fat Pound Cake 254

Maple Spice Cake 256
Old Fashioned Strawberry
   Shortcake 257
Pear Crumble Cake 258
Sweet Potato Snack Cake 259
Candy
  Peanut Butter Fudge
    Crunchy Snack 247
Cookies
  Brownies 260
  Chocolate Oatmeal Jumbles 261
  Chocolate Raspberry Treats 262
  Colossal Chocolate Chippers 263
  Cranberry Spice Cookies 264
  Fudge Frosted Oatmeal Cookies 265
  Fudgy Cocoa Brownies 266
  Georgia's Fudge Bars 267
  Great Pumpkin Cookies 268
  Light and Luscious Brownies 269
  Oatmeal Raisin Cookies 270
  Sugar-Free Oatmeal Cookies 271
  Sweetie Bars 272
  The Best Cake Brownies 273
  Thumbprint Cookies 274
  Ultimate Oatmeal Cookies 275
  Whole Wheat Chocolate Chippers ... 276
Frostings
  Fluffy Maple Frosting 277
  Luscious Lemon Sauce 278
Honey Cheese Crepes 244
Maple-Glazed Apple Slices 245
Old Fashioned Bread Pudding 246
Pies and Pastry
  Apple Pie 279
  Banana Cream Pie 280
  Crunchy Cereal Pie Crust 281
  Key Lime Pie 282
  Lemon Chess Pie 283
  Meringue 284
  Pecan Pie 285

Pumpkin Pie 286
Sugar Free Pecan Pudding Pie 287
Dill Dip 23
Dill Salmon Salad 91
Duo of Grilled Squash 207

E

Easy Gazpacho 70
Easy Lasagna 116
Egg Salad Sandwiches 130

F

Fat Free Creamy Cucumber Dressing 107
Fat-Free French Bread 50
Fat-Free Matzo Balls 71
Fettuccine Alfredo 117
Fettuccine with Shrimp 154
Florentine Frittata 208
Flounder Baked in Lettuce Leaves 155
Fluffy Maple Frosting 277
Focaccia 51
Focaccia Sandwiches 131
French Onion Soup 72
Fresh Glazed Beets 209
Fudge Frosted Oatmeal Cookies 265
Fudgy Cocoa Brownies 266

G

Garlic Bread 53
Gazpacho Soup 73
Georgia's Fudge Bars 267
German Cucumber Salad 92
Ginger Grilled Fish 156
Gingered Carrots 210
Gingered Dijon Salmon 157
Grape Salad 93
Great Pumpkin Cookies 268
Green Bean Salad 94
Green Beans with Toasted Pecans 211
Green Pea and Blue Cheese Salad 95

Green Pea and Rice Salad 96
Green Rice 118
Grilled Hoagie Sandwiches 132
Grilled Marinated Chicken 184
Grilled Potatoes 213
Grilled Vegetables 212
Guacamole 24

H

Ham and Lima Bean Stew 74
Ham with Cabbage and Apples 168
Hamburger Soup 75
Heart Healthy Oriental
      Chicken and Vegetables 185
Hearty Beef Casserole 143
Herbed Pot Roast 144
Herbed Vinigrette 108
Honey Cheese Crepes 244
Honey Mustard Dip 25
Hot and Spicy Tomato Salsa 26
Hot Bean Dip 27
Hot Crab Dip 28

I

Italian Baked Halibut 158
Italian Fish in Foil Packets 159
Italian Style Green Beans 214

J

Jicama and Citrus Salad 97

K

Key Lime Pie 282

L

Lamb with Garlic and Rosemary 164
Lamb with Mint Sauce 165
Lean(er) Pesto Sauce with Pasta 119
Lemon Chess Pie 283
Lemon-Pineapple Chicken 186

Light and Luscious Brownies 269
Low-fat Pound Cake 254
Luscious Lemon Sauce 278

M

Main Dishes
  Pork and Ham
      Ham with Cabbage and Apples 168
      Pork Chops in Apple Juice 169
Maple Baked Beans 215
Maple Spice Cake 255
Maple-Glazed Apple Slices 245
Marinated Broccoli 216
Meat Dishes
  Beef
      Beef and Cornbread Casserole 141
      Beef in Mushroom Sauce 142
      Hearty Beef Casserole 143
      Herbed Pot Roast 144
      Microwave Meatloaf 145
      Peppered Beef Tenderloin 146
      Stuffed Cabbage 147
      Veal and Apple Scaloppine 148
      Veal and Fettucine Florentine 149
  Fish and Seafood
      Baked Fish With Vegetables 150
      Baked Halibut 151
      Broiled Sole with Cheese 152
      Broiled Swordfish with Mango Salsa 153
      Fettuccine with Shrimp 154
      Flounder Baked in Lettuce Leaves ... 155
      Ginger Grilled Fish 156
      Gingered Dijon Salmon 157
      Italian Baked Halibut 158
      Italian Fish in Foil Packets 159
      Poached Sole with Tarragon 160
      Scallops with Roasted Red
          Pepper Coulis 161
      Shrimp Quesadillas 162
      Stuffed Red Snapper 163

Lamb
- Lamb with Garlic and Rosemary 164
- Lamb with Mint Sauce 165
- Pecan Crusted Lamb Chops 166

Pork and Ham
- Black Bean and Pork Stew 167
- Pork with Creamy Basil Sauce 170
- South Seas Casserole 171
- Sweet and Sour Pork Chops 172

Poultry
- Apricot-Baked Chicken 173
- Chicken and Apples Over Fettucini . 174
- Chicken Cacciatore 175
- Chicken Dijon 176
- Chicken Divan 177
- Chicken Fajitas 178
- Chicken Garlic Sticks 179
- Chicken Pomodoro 180
- Chicken Roasted with Rosemary and Garlic 181
- Chicken with Pesto 182
- Curried Chicken 183
- Grilled Marinated Chicken 184
- Heart Healthy Oriental Chicken and Vegetables 185
- Lemon-Pineapple Chicken 186
- Orange Chicken Stir-Fry 187
- Paella 188
- Pasta with Chicken and Peas 189
- Rosemary and Lemon Chicken 190
- Salsa Baked Chicken 191
- Spicy Indian Chicken 192
- Spicy Oven Fried Drumsticks 193

Melon Soup for Summer 76
Meringue 284
Mexican Layer Dip 29
Microwave Meatloaf 145
Mocha Fudge Cake 256
Mushroom Barley 217
Mushroom Barley Soup 77
Mushroom Cheese Sandwich 133
Mushrooms Florentine 30

N

Nacho Cheese Dip 31
Nutty Wheat Bread 54

O

Oatmeal Raisin Cookies 270
Old Fashioned Bread Pudding 246
Old Fashioned Strawberry Shortcake 257
Onion Cheese Puffs 32
Onion Spread 32
Orange Chicken Stir-Fry 187
Oriental Dressing 109
Oven Zucchini Fries 33

P

Paella 188

Pasta
- Baked Pasta Primavera 113
- Creamy Linguini 115
- Easy Lasagna 116
- Fettuccine Alfredo 117
- Lean(er) Pesto Sauce with Pasta 119
- Pasta Shells Stuffed With Cheeses 120
- Pasta with Fresh Tomatoes 121
- Pasta with Pine Nut Garlic Sauce 122

Pasta Shells Stuffed With Cheeses 120
Pasta with Chicken and Peas 189
Pasta with Fresh Tomatoes 121
Pasta with Pine Nut Garlic Sauce 122
Peach Perfect Muffins 55
Peanut Butter Fudge Crunchy Snack 247
Pear Crumble Cake 258

Peas with Mint 218
Pecan Crusted Lamb Chops 166
Pecan Pie 285
Pepper Cheese Dip 34
Peppered Beef Tenderloin 146
Pita Pizzas 56
Poached Sole with Tarragon 160
Pork Chops in Apple Juice 169
Pork with Creamy Basil Sauce 170
Portobello Mushroom Sandwiches 134
Potato Cheese Casserole 219
Potato Chowder 78
Potato Gratin 220
Pretzels 57
Pumpkin Pie 286

Q

Quick Pasta Salad 99

R

Red Potato Casserole 221
Rice
    Brown Rice with Vegetables 114
    Green Rice 118
    Rice Pilaf 123
    Risotto 124
    Saffron Rice and Black Beans 125
Rice Pilaf 123
Risotto 124
Roasted Corn Relish 222
Roasted Corn y Salsa Pita Sandwiches 135
Rosemary and Lemon Chicken 190

S

Saffron Rice and Black Beans 125
Salad Dressings

Blue Cheese Dressing 105
Buttermilk Herb Dressing 106
Fat Free Creamy Cucumber Dressing .. 107
Herbed Vinigrette 108
Oriental Dressing 109
Salads
    Cheddar Pea Salad 87
    Chicken Salad 88
    Corn and Bean Salad 89
    Corn Relish 98
    Crab or Shrimp Salad 90
    Dill Salmon Salad 91
    German Cucumber Salad 92
    Grape Salad 93
    Green Bean Salad 94
    Green Pea and Blue Cheese Salad 95
    Green Pea and Rice Salad 96
    Jicama and Citrus Salad 97
    Quick Pasta Salad 99
    Savory Broccoli Potato Salad 100
    Spinach and Chicken Salad 101
    Spinach Salad 102
    Spinach Salad with Curried Dressing .. 103
    Tabbouleh 104
Salmon Tortilla Appetizers 35
Salsa Baked Chicken 191
Sandwiches
    Chicken and Avocado Sandwich 129
    Egg Salad Sandwiches 130
    Focaccia Sandwiches 131
    Grilled Hoagie Sandwiches 132
    Mushroom Cheese Sandwich 133
    Portobello Mushroom Sandwiches 134
    Roasted Corn y Salsa Pita Sandwiches 135
    Seafood Salad Sandwich 136
    Veggie Pita Sandwiches 137
Savory Broccoli Potato Salad 100
Savory Potato Casserole 223

Scallops with Roasted
    Red Pepper Coulis 161
Seafood Salad Sandwich 136
Sesame Broccoli 224
Shrimp Quesadillas 162
Soups
    Bean and Cabbage Soup 63
    Chicken Corn Chowder 66
    Chicken-flavored Vegetable Soup 67
    Cream of Onion Soup 68
    Cream of Vegetable Soup 69
    Easy Gazpacho 70
    Fat-Free Matzo Balls 71
    French Onion Soup 72
    Gazpacho Soup 73
    Hamburger Soup 75
    Melon Soup for Summer 76
    Mushroom Barley Soup 77
    Potato Chowder 78
    Southwestern Black Bean Soup 79
    Tortilla Soup 80
    Tuna Chowder 81
    Vegetable Soup 82
    Yogurt Soup for a Hot Day 84
South Seas Casserole 171
Southwestern Black Bean Soup 79
Spaghetti Squash Marinara 225
Spicy Indian Chicken 192
Spicy Oven Fried Drumsticks 193
Spinach and Cheese Bites 36
Spinach and Chicken Salad 101
Spinach Dip 37
Spinach Dip 2 38
Spinach Pancakes 226
Spinach Salad 102
Spinach Salad with Curried Dressing 103
Stews
    Bean and Pasta Stew 64
    Black Bean Chili 65

Ham and Lima Bean Stew 74
    Vegetarian Chili 83
Stir Fried Vegetables 227
Strawberry Oatmeal Muffins 58
Stuffed Artichokes 228
Stuffed Bell Peppers 229
Stuffed Cabbage 147
Stuffed Mushrooms 39
Stuffed Red Snapper 163
Sugar Free Pecan Pudding Pie 287
Sugar Free Sticky Buns 59
Sugar-Free Oatmeal Cookies 271
Summer Squash Noodles 230
Sweet and Sour Pork Chops 172
Sweet Glazed Carrots 231
Sweet Potato Casserole 232
Sweet Potato Snack Cake 259
Sweetie Bars 272

T

Tabbouleh 104
Tamale Balls 40
The Best (and Easiest) Green
    Beans You Will Ever E 233
The Best 7 layer Mexican Dip 41
The Best Cake Brownies 273
Thumbprint Cookies 274
Tomato-Mozzarella Bites 42
Tomatoes Stuffed with Salmon 43
Tortilla Roll-Ups 44
Tortilla Soup 80
Tuna Chowder 81

U

Ultimate Oatmeal Cookies 275

V

Veal and Apple Scaloppine 148

Veal and Fettucine Florentine 149
Vegetable Casserole 234
Vegetable Dip with Zip 45
Vegetable Pizza Crust 60
Vegetable Quesadillas 46
Vegetable Soup 82
Vegetables
    Asparagus Torta 197
    Baked Acorn Squash 198
    Balsamic Marinated Vegetables 199
    Boiled Parslied New Potatoes 200
    Broccoli with Pearl Onions Casserole .. 201
    Broiled Tomatoes with Horseradish 202
    Buttermilk Mashed Potatoes 203
    Cabbage Casserole 204
    Chili Topped Potatoes 205
    Creamy Green Beans 206
    Duo of Grilled Squash 207
    Florentine Frittata 208
    Fresh Glazed Beets 209
    Gingered Carrots 210
    Green Beans with Toasted Pecans 211
    Grilled Potatoes 213
    Grilled Vegetables 212
    Italian Style Green Beans 214
    Maple Baked Beans 215
    Marinated Broccoli 216
    Mushroom Barley 217
    Peas with Mint 218
    Potato Cheese Casserole 219
    Potato Gratin 220
    Red Potato Casserole 221
    Roasted Corn Relish 222
    Savory Potato Casserole 223
    Sesame Broccoli 224
    Spaghetti Squash Marinara 225
    Spinach Pancakes 226
    Stir Fried Vegetables 227
    Stuffed Artichokes 228
    Stuffed Bell Peppers 229
    Summer Squash Noodles 230
    Sweet Glazed Carrots 231
    Sweet Potato Casserole 232
    The Best (and Easiest) Green
        Beans You Will Ever E 233
    Vegetable Casserole 234
    Vegetarian Moussaka 235
    Zucchini Casserole 236
    Zucchini Casserole Special 237
Vegetarian Chili 83
Vegetarian Moussaka 235
Veggie Pita Sandwiches 137

W

Whole Wheat Chocolate Chippers 276

Y

Yogurt Soup for a Hot Day 84

Z

Zucchini Casserole 236
Zucchini Casserole Special 237